Natural VISION *Improvement*

JANET GOODRICH Ph.D

Janet grew up in the farming country of mid-Michigan in the US. She spent her primary grades in an old one-room red brick schoolhouse where the same teacher fostered her growth for seven years. At the age of seven she was given a pair of eyeglasses for myopia and astigmatism and wore them constantly for the next 20 years. Secondary school was in a small village followed by four years at the University of Michigan where she learned languages, philosophy, and behavioral psychology. A year was spent in Berlin on a Fulbright scholarship and another year teaching high school in her home town. Then came an abrupt change of life and pace. She moved to Southern California in 1967 and became involved in Reichian therapy, natural childbirth, alternative education and the Bates Method. After shedding her glasses she completed training as a Reichian therapist which she practised for ten years. This work has evolved into seminars in eyesight and emotional healing. She designed and built a wholistic health centre in Los Angeles which was home for natural vision improvement, chiropractic and nutritional counseling. Her Ph.D in psychology was on eyesight and character. After a lecture tour to Australia in 1980 she decided to explore the strong personal 'dreaming' experience of that occasion by residing 'down under'. From there she continues to transmit the lore of natural vision by training instructors in the US, Europe and Australia.

Blink, Yawn, Palm, Sunning
For - Wear   Massage Neck
Swinging

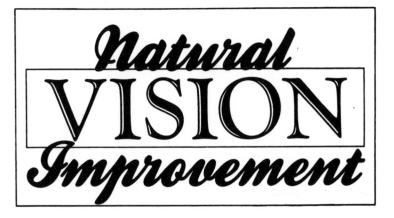

Natural VISION Improvement

JANET GOODRICH

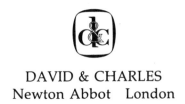

DAVID & CHARLES
Newton Abbot   London

British Library Cataloguing in Publication Data

Goodrich, Janet
    Natural vision improvement.
    1. Vision disorders—Treatment
    2. Self-care, Health
    I. Title
    617.7'068   RE61

    ISBN 0-7153-9019-8

Designed by Leonie Stott
Illustration by Louise Coutts
Typeset by Trade Graphics Pty Ltd

Printed in Great Britain
by Butler & Tanner Limited, Frome and London
for David & Charles Publishers plc
Brunel House   Newton Abbot   Devon

This book is for my mother,
Mildred Devereaux Goodrich.

ACKNOWLEDGEMENTS

My appreciation for learning and encouragement goes to Philip Curcuruto, Charles Thompson, Deena Metzgar, Harriet Machado, Charles Kelley, Meroe Sommers, Paul Dennison, Raymond Gottlieb, Hans Friend, Ken Chenery, Paul Reps, Hilda Reach, Ian Niven, Beth Bolton, Lorna Seabrook, Laura Sewell, Sara Estep, Gary Robb, Jorge Calderon, Shiela Posner, Frances Guerin, Keith Millar, Kara Hanson-Millar, Wolfgang Gillessen, Doreen Cott, Cybele, Carina, Travis and Jeff, to all my students and student-teachers. Special gratitude to my illustrators, Richard Montoya and Louise Coutts.

The author and publishers wish to thank Plenum Publishing Corporation, N.Y. for permission to reproduce figures on pages 7 and 52, from Alfred Yarbus, *Eye Movements and Vision*, 1973.

Contents

Preface

Vision is important to all of us. When it becomes unbalanced, blurred, unhealthy, we want to be able to do something about it. This book provides an avenue for you to travel on — a journey in which you can learn about and renew your total visual functioning. Many people's desires for better eyesight are concentrated in the wish to rid themselves of their glasses. This is possible. Thousands have accomplished it to the bewilderment of optometrists and eye doctors over the last several decades. To many eye doctors, the prescription of corrective lenses has been the only means to deal with blurred vision. The wearing of glasses is meant to compensate or 'correct' myopia (blur in the distance), hyperopia (blur up close), astigmatism (a warp in the front surface of the eyeball or in the lens which causes blur at all distances). Then we have presbyopia or 'old age sight' where the lens stiffens and grows slightly larger with age. This condition, which is preventable with a bit of knowledge and action, is not as inevitable as we have been led to believe. To be sure, we may grow generally less pliable with age, yet to succumb to the crutch of reading glasses leads to rapid deterioration of the tone and fitness of the eyes. The conditions of squint, or wall eyes caused by chronically tight eye muscles which pull and hold the eyes into positions of high stress can also be alleviated by natural means. Sometimes after years of wearing glasses or not using an eye as in amblyopia, certain areas of the brain require an awakening. This reactivation of the brain accompanies the renewal of vision.

Many benefits are to be derived from nurturing your own visual process. These have to do with release of stress, better visual functioning in the areas of learning, coordination, and even relief of the pain and discomfort that often stems from unbalanced eyesight. It is also possible to adapt the activities presented in this book to your family and work situations where eyesight habits are imitated and expressed, where the effects of your environment take their toll on your vision (such as lighting, video and computer use, etc). So, whether you use glasses or not, this book is for everybody. Its ideas are to be used everywhere. The whole visual world provides the materials.

The text has been designed sequentially, building a fresh set of habits to replace the old. Yet it is also possible to delve into any part of the book as you are inclined. One day you may want to refine your ability to visualize, another time you may feel like polishing acuity. Specific programs are given for those who feel most secure with a pattern to follow. At the same time you are encouraged to understand the principles underlying the activities so that you will come to the point where you are able to put together your own program, blending it with your particular lifestyle and ambitions/pastimes.

reading the text, you come to any terms you do not understand be sure to consult the glossary at the end of the book.

Results YOU can create for the physical are:
1. Better visual acuity to the point of not needing eyeglasses.
2. Coordination of the eyes at all distances.
3. Increased speed of perception.
4. Higher color perception and awareness.
5. Prevention of visual blur.
6. Increased depth perception.
7. Encouragement of the normal self-healing process of the body.

Possible results on other levels include:
1. Increased ability to learn by activating the right (visual) hemisphere of the brain.
2. Higher intellect (connective and analytic abilities) as the left hemisphere gets help from visualizing.
3. A more active memory based on visual images.
4 Communication lines broaden as you build your confidence to talk to people through your eyes.
5. Creativity and confidence grow as you start nurturing your own well-being and imaginaton.

The changing of vision can be a spiritual adventure as well if you wish to expand your seeing in all directions from the physical to the eternal, from outer vision to inner vision.

Chapter 1

Natural Vision is Ours to Keep

Natural vision is seeing with every part of ourselves. From our physical eyes right through our feelings, thoughts, dreams, creative insights, and spiritual unfolding, vision permeates all our life experiences. And it is ours to keep.

If we regard vision in this broadened wholistic way it gives us the doorway, the inspiration and the knowledge to maintain and improve our seeing ability. If vision is all these inter-related parts, we might ask 'Why must it only roll downhill and then be irretrievable? Don't we have within us somewhere the power not only to recover and maintain our eyesight, but also to develop it even further?' There we stand, scratching our heads, either straining through glasses, or fending them off, muttering, 'There must be a better way'.

Fortunately for those of us who want our visual experience to be progressive throughout our life, to be full of excitement and beauty, replete with 'aha' and 'I see that clearly now', there are answers. We are able to keep, improve, develop and expand our vision through our own actions.

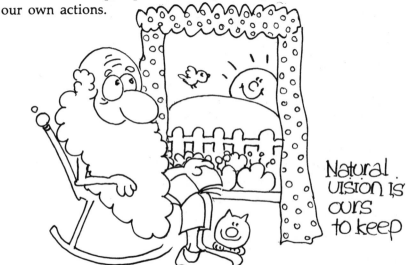

Natural vision is ours to keep

The maturing of the 20th century has brought with it gifts from many areas of orthodox research and unorthodox experimentation. To improve our vision naturally we will draw from both the narrowed eye of science and the open-minded approach of alternative medical pioneers, William H. Bates and Wilhelm Reich. These brilliant physicians moved beyond their conventional training to theorize and teach about the mind/body connection early in this century. Despite unremitting derision from entrenched professional interests their sensible and useful ideas were acknowledged and spread by alternative healers and teachers.

Natural vision improvement stems more from experiencing the vital connectiveness of human life and human sight, than from pursuing a rigid program of ritualized eye exercises. It takes the widest possible view of sight and recognizes that the impetus for improvement may come from any facet of the total visual experience. The improvement you will find in your sight comes primarily from your increasing capacity for aliveness. Basic life energy will pulsate through your mind and body resulting in sparkling expressive eyes and revived visual clarity.

The challenge of bettering eyesight is yours alone, sight being a particularly intimate and personal phenomenon. You are the one who accepts the challenge and makes the changes. And you receive the credit. Improving vision naturally is an internal transformation, not a treatment, cure, or makeover by external forces.

The confidence generated by ameliorating your vision *to any extent* adds to the loving of yourself, the world and others. With these ideas in sight let's begin our exploration of the natural vision concepts with an experience in *seeing*.

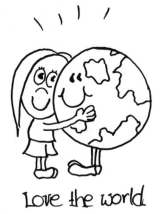

Love the world

NATURAL VISION IS BEAUTY, ENERGY, ALIVENESS

A small window in the upper storey of an old granary in Austria opens out to a lush green meadow. The wind dances through the trailing branches of the birch trees. It is spring. Occasionally a flock of tender white petals wafts past the window. Pollen-laden bees weave a buzzy cape over the apple tree. A wave of air scented with deep purple lilacs pours through the room. Alive beauty is rampant in the sunwarmed hills. I see it in myriad ways, I perceive each glowing burst of color, each manifestation of life energy with my eyes. Does this mean that I am equally as alive? I ponder the relationship between the seer and the seen. Am I a bee, an apple blossom, a flexible branch in the moment that I take in and form their images in my mind? Are my eyes as lively and brimming with energy as what I see? I'm aware that they are now loose, flexible, happy as I move my attention across the nodding burgundy clover

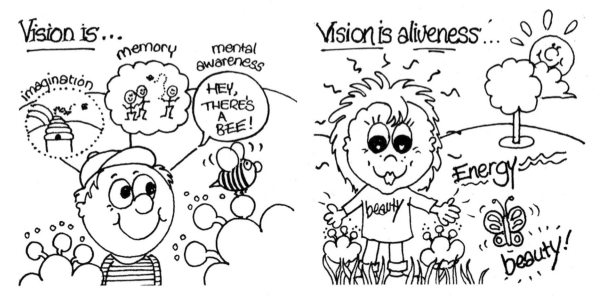

and the shimmering buttercups in the sea of greenness below. What a joy it is to be seeing, to have a visual system that responds so fully to the changing and harmonious kaleidoscope of life taking place around me.

NATURAL VISION IS MENTAL ATTENTION, IMAGINATION, MEMORY

The sky darkens. The trees pause in their swaying to attend the thunder that tumbles through the spacious atmosphere. I listen. My mind wants a reference. Ah! It sounds like the aluminium sheeting on Woden's roof is rattling. A black and gold puff buzzes through the open window and slouches in a crevice on the pine wall, discontented at this imminent dampening of its floral feast. I pay attention to the rain. The drops fall straight down, echoing the stance of the slim fir trees. As a child I was able to easily write stories when thunderstorms raged. The images came into my mind and I put them on paper as the day's energy huddled under a moist grey blanket. I realize now the role of my inner-picture making, my imagination. What I experienced in childhood I carry with me. Those memory images blend with the present. I see in the present with the help of the past which lingers in my nervous system, in my brain. The raindrops become more distinct as I recall those early sensory experiences — walking home from school through a grey-white sheen, tasting the bright coolness on my lips, the crisp scent of wet vegetation in my nose. The cleansing rain sluiced over my yellow slicker and trickled down the back of my neck.

The window swings itself closed in a sudden gust. The latch rocks. I am inwardly activated, excited. The world is inviting me to respond, to participate more and more in the seeing of itself through me. The past, the future are gathered in now to energize and clarify the seeing of the present. Thunder bellows again, trailing itself out after a long exhalation. The carpet below glows emerald. Rainwater tea quivers in the lacquered buttercups. A short-lived storm, sunlight soon lifts up the shower curtain. I imagine there is a rainbow somewhere, arching over the undulating hills. I inhale deeply and feel grateful for this unique place and the living gifts of nature. I am confident that I am able to be involved in this marvellous mix of inner and outer joy, to affect the quality of my vision by choice. I am able to share and support this way of seeing in others. I walk out the barn door. A rainbow gives me a colorful upside-down smile.

THE OPTION TO WITHDRAW

I could curtail my vision right now. I could sit at the window and take myself somewhere else, into worries about my family far away, to concerns about money, into a fantasy that doesn't harmonize with the world around me. I could ignore the flowers, the creatures, the sounds. Withdrawal of my perception is my current choice. I could eat sugar all day and end up in a daze with dizzy eyes. I could decide the countryside is boring and engross myself in a best seller for hours. I could think that other people are uninterested in me and avoid their eyes. I used to do all these things. For twenty years opting out in these ways was habitual for me. Thick lenses sat upon my nose correcting my vision that was obscured by myopia and astigmatism. Trapped in a diminished perspective of life and self, often my world appeared two-dimensional and grey. I did my best to compensate. I got outdoors, exercised, took chances, had adventures. Still, I lived with an inner tension that I learned to hide even from myself. Wide-open and unfamiliar places gave me a feeling of queasiness. My eyes squinted through the thick glass. My neck and shoulders were stiff. Although I did well enough academically I wasn't satisfied with high grades given for correct regurgitation of ideas that had been fed to me. Mentally and physically I felt like I wanted to burst free — from what? I didn't know.

All that has changed now. The depression has been replaced by skills for maintaining and expressing optimism. I paint and write and create my life with enthusiasm. I have not worn glasses since 1969. Through the ideas of Dr Wilhelm Reich I learned to understand the unconscious holding back of life energy in the eyes, the perceptual blur and the odd awkward feelings that this constriction generates.

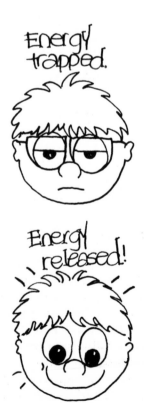

Energy trapped.

Energy released!

In his book *Character Analysis* Reich pointed out: 'What one feels is not the armoring itself but only the *distortion of perception of life*.' Armoring refers to our total defensive stance including rigidities of personality and chronically tight muscles which hold back emotions. The armored person becomes 'empty' (there are few images in the mind). The protected part of the body is 'rigid' (unable to shift attention). The armoring that exists in the visual system is physically manifested as 'a contraction and immobilization of all or most of the muscles of the eyeball, lids, forehead and tear glands'. The mental reaction to the unused tear glands is the resolve never to show weakness by crying. This holding in the eyes does not change into another static state — of frozen 20/20 clarity after being released. Vision follows the natural rhythm of all living beings. It rises and falls, intensifies and wanes, in its response to our engagement with external and internal environments. This theme of pulsation in vision will be looked at again in regard to children (chapter 10) and the integration of right and left hemispheres of the brain (chapter 12). During illness, negative emotional states, and fatigue, the visual energy may abate and perception diminish for a time. But it is never lost. Reopening and encouraging this natural pulse of vision whether one wears glasses or not will result in a lovely reawakening of your whole personality and being.

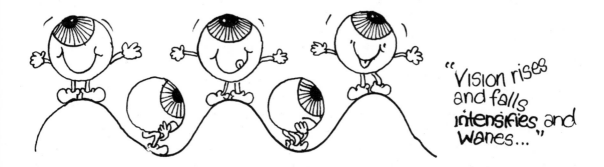

"Vision rises and falls intensifies and wanes..."

THE PHYSICAL EYE

Yes, visual blur is manifested in the physical eye. Yet when we consider the physical we are observing only one end of the human visual system. It is the tip of the iceberg. To deny all the accompanying facets of vision limits our capacity to alter the physical. We are usually taught that the eye is a 'camera' composed of a set of muscles, nerves and optical components that receive light, transpose the incoming stimulation into nerve impulses which are transmitted to the visual brain or cortex where 'vision' occurs. The role of the total being, the rest of the brain and personal adaptations to life, are ignored.

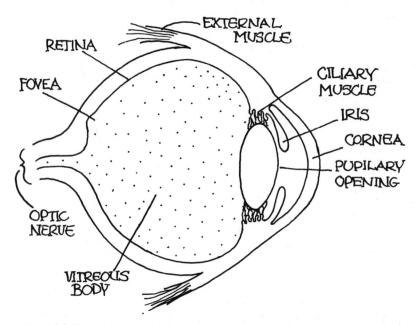

Arnold Gesell, who did brilliant studies of the development of children and their vision said, 'Seeing is not a separate isolated function, it is profoundly integrated with the total action system of the child — his posture, his manual skills and coordination, his intelligence and his personality. He sees with his whole being.' Gesell was aware of the pitfalls of an over-simplistic analogy: 'The metaphor of the camera has tended to obscure ... significant developmental changes.'

We are told that physical answers are all that's needed for a purely physical problem. Therefore a pair of compensatory lenses ground to the state of our visual system at the moment of examination in the eye practitioner's office is placed on our noses. There has been an ever increasing percentage of the population of many countries turning up with refractive errors: myopia, astigmatism and squint (turned eyes). Prescribing glasses has not stemmed this tide nor cast any light on the causes of the lowering vision of so many of us.

Behavioral optometrists often use training glasses with children to offset the early development of myopia in school. And they advocate glasses for preschool children as a possible means of preventing amblyopia (lazy eye). A very few of the more progressive thinkers in this group will admit that even myopia is changeable. Why? Because of their own experience, or because someone entered their office with a history of myopia and read the eyechart without glasses at a level way beyond the expected medical incapacity. Sometimes this improvement in a condition considered officially

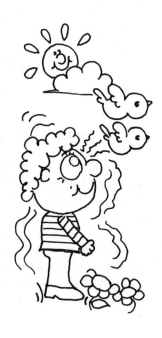

'hopeless' or 'physically impossible' is confirmed by objective examination of the eye (retinoscopy). Usually, however, there was no observable change in the axial length of the eye and the remarkable subjective performance was termed 'reinterpretation of the blur' — a statement meant to discredit the reality of the clarity the patient experienced and the natural method by which he or she had achieved his or her new perception. The natural methods used by these people may have been the Bates Method, nutrition, yoga, chiropractic, or in some cases simple prayer. Human potential has a habit of leapfrogging over established, authorized pronouncements and predictions.

IS THERE A CHANCE FOR ME?

You might say, 'Janet improved her sight and so did those other folk whose names I see in the back of this book, but that doesn't mean it's going to work for me.' My response to this statement of self-doubt is 'No, it does not work for you or anyone.' This way of putting things reflects the policy of the last hundred years of giving away our responsibility for health, lifestyle and well-being into the hands of experts and outside forces. This doesn't mean we are not to consult and utilize those learned and experienced friends. It simply is to point out the often sneaky and unconscious attitude that the crucial changes in our life come from outside. We will be treated, cured, pummeled, shaken, analyzed, doped, worked for and on, made over by an external agent more knowing than we ourselves.

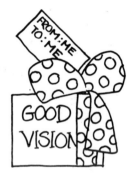

It is indeed a great challenge and not necessarily the rose-strewn path to pick up the prerogatives for your own life, particularly where there is fear and threat and ignorance. Yet the rewards for doing so are extensive and significant. If your eyesight improves, eyestrain lessens, or you feel more comfortable in any way in your life as a result of absorbing and activating the information in this book, use your own hand to pat your own back.

OPENING THE DOOR

Nature gave us the capacity for clear vision and also the means of restoring it after it has been 'lost'. Given some sound knowledge, personal encouragement and support you have the option to recreate your vision for yourself, at least to 'give it a go'. Desire and a receptive attitude count more than age, history and degree of blur. It takes heart to face up to the 'can't do that!' whether it is voiced by others or by oneself. The benefits of improving your vision naturally are many, including self-confidence, more enjoyment of life and often the appearance of unsuspected creative abilities. As you recover and develop your visual capacity you will release a great deal of

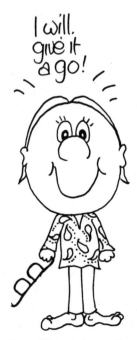

Natural Vision is Ours to Keep

Vision is...

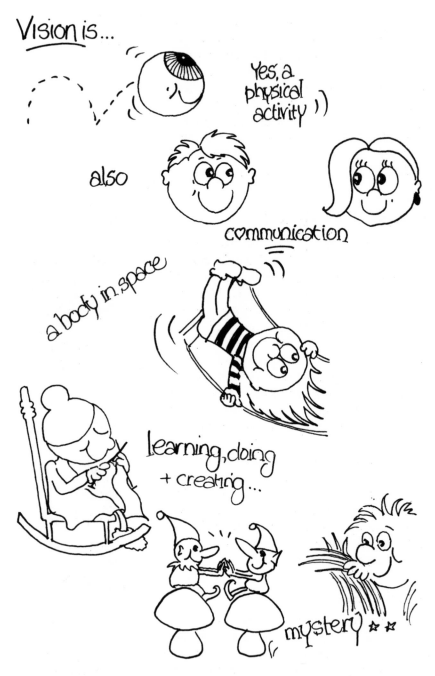

Yes, a physical activity

also

communication

a body in space

learning, doing + creating...

mystery ✦ ✦

energy. These surges of energy that come with increased perception, may seem scary or too thrilling at times. You are experiencing the tidal pulses of your own lifestream. You will be able to flow with this strong rhythm even through the rough currents. Ending up with pleasure in self you will have faced your own inertia (resistance to change) and refound your art of seeing.

Natural Vision Improvement

TAKE A STEP

In the next two chapters we will consider the psychological aspects of visual distortions. To this we add activities garnered from my seventeen years of teaching vision improvement inspired by the ideas of Dr Bates and his follower Margaret Corbett who developed many practical vision games during the 1930s to the 1950s in her School of Eye Education in Los Angeles. I have adapted both their work to today's setting and lifestyles. Some technical data is presented so that our minds have the relevant facts concerning anatomy and physiology. We then blend in the latest theories of whole brain functioning and self-healing. I encourage you to use this whole book in a creative and personal fashion.

Both you and I know that reading a book is not the thing itself. The original Bates book, which has been selling consistently since its publication in 1921, has gathered dust on many bookshelves. Yet the fact that people continue to buy it reveals the basic urge towards seeing perfectly without glasses is strong and ongoing. Translating the messages given in this book into action will brighten your mind and vision. Robotically repeating eye exercises (a left-brain action) does not stimulate that part of you that is essentially visual — your imaginative, relaxing, harmonizing aspect (the right-brain contribution). Vision is a continuous, in the moment, creation of your whole being. Take daring leaps and do your best. Know that we are using the following:

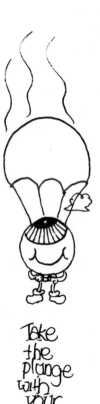

Take the plunge with your vision

knowledge
self-responsibility
the interrelationship of body, mind and spirit
games and good humor
visualization
supportive positive attitude
in a format that is:
adaptable to your lifestyle
flexible
effective
maintainable
sensual and fun.

Chapter 2

Transforming the Myopic Character

THE MYOPIA PUZZLE

At age thirteen, I read an article in a national magazine on eyesight. If you are far-sighted, I learned, your eyes *might* improve and you won't always have to wear glasses. However, if you are near-sighted your eyes will never change.

I sat there on the couch in the farmhouse stunned, feeling condemned. What was it about me behind my thick myopic glasses that meant I couldn't jump on a trampoline, climb mountains, run across the fields without fear of breaking or losing my awkward spectacles.

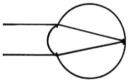

normal
eyeball

The answer to my question evaded me until, at twenty-four years of age, I lay on another couch breathing life back into myself. My Reichian therapist, Dr Phillip Curcuruto, who was guiding my reacquaintance with life energy, said to me, 'Someday you will want to get rid of those things'. He was shaking the heavy glasses I kept so close to me at all times. I certainly agreed but had never found a glimmer of possibility in this notion. However, over the next two years hints and bits of the myopic puzzle fell into my hands. First, the thinking patterns that lay behind that magazine article come to light and I learned why prospective students still say to me today, 'But how can I change my myopia? My doctor says it is impossible because my eyeball is too long.' 'Yes,' I reply, 'It's true that your eyeball *may* be too long, but that is not the end of the story.'

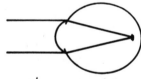

elongated
myopic eyeball

During the last 130 years, an array of causative factors underlying the myopia due to an elongation of the eyeballs, or refractive myopia where the eyeball has a normal length, have been considered by vision researchers. There is still, today, no common agreement on the cause of myopia or the way to alleviate it. The prescribing of glasses and contact lenses or the highly questionable surgery, radial keratotomy, do not reach nor alter the source of myopia.

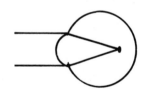

normal eyeball
with refractive
myopia

In order to understand from a consumer's point of view the discordance we might encounter in the professionals' marketplace, let's look at the following chart.

Chart 1

Practitioners	General Opinion on Myopia	General Response to Myopia	Action Usually Taken
Ophthalmologists: Medical doctors, licensed to: examine eyes and visual function prescribe compensatory lenses prescribe drugs, use surgery diagnose and treat pathological conditions	A fixed, anatomical and physiological condition, incurable, causes are inherited or unknown	It stays the same, It worsens, or It doesn't improve	Prescribe compensatory lenses or use radial keratotomy
Optometrists: Licensed to: examine eyes and visual function prescribe compensatory lenses diagnose pathological conditions	Same as above	Same as above	Prescribe compensatory lenses.
Vision therapists 'Behavioral optometrists': Optometrists trained to: give eye exercises treat anomalies of visual function	Causes are environmental stress, over-use of close-point, adaptation to modern day lifestyles	'Perhaps myopia can be halted' (this group in the U.S. is officially disdainful of the 'unproven' Bates Method)	Same as above and some often give plus lenses to myopic school children to relieve the stress of over-accomodation for near tasks, to prevent the onset of myopia, halt its progress, or improve it
Wholistic vision therapists: Optometrists who perform all of the above plus discussing and utilizing the Bates Method, yoga, autogenic training, nutrition, chiropractic, etc.	Same as above and acknowledge psychological involvement with myopia	Myopia can be improved	Prescribe and often reduce the strength of compensatory lenses. In addition, attend to total being and environmental factors. View eyesight as a self-correctable system. Open to the beneficial activities stemming from the Bates method
Psychologists: If clinically licensed, they work with various methods to transmute or transcend emotional factors	No general viewpoint	No organized response	There are many individual research projects delving into causative factors of myopia
Lay practitioners: Unlicenced teachers of wholistic approaches. Unsanctioned by established interests. Bates Method teachers, Natural Vision instructors, and individualists who have taught relaxation, imagery, stress reduction, in non-medical, non-optometric ways	All states of refractive error, including myopia can be changed for the better	Teach individuals and groups in private homes, wholistic health centres, schools, and businesses	Using verbal communication, music, imagination, and caring, eclectic modalities, people are taught how to improve their own sight

A SOCIOLOGIST'S VIEW

In 1981, as part of his certified training as a natural vision instructor, sociology professor Raymond Welch wrote an intriguing thesis on the cultural and social factors bearing upon the rise of myopia in America. Rather than viewing humans as naive recipients of the insensitive bombardment of the industrial revolution, Professor Welch points out that *something* had been chosen to defeat the conditions of natural vision. Certain morals were internalized which shaped the personal psychology of Americans for the ensuing 200 years of increasing estrangement from nature and self and the ultimate homolateral 'left-brain' emphasis which we are just now learning to heal. The circumstantial indications that Welch considers are:

1. The modern optical industry began in the 1780s and spectacle manufacturing became big business in the 1800s.
2. Prominent leaders began to appear in public and portraiture in metal-framed spectacles (today, notice how the wearing of glasses by child or adult in advertising connotes scholarliness, responsibility, and intelligent performance).
3. The influence of Benjamin Franklin, inventor of bifocals and moral idealist, in the fields of commerce, law and education. Franklin was obsessed with an orderly existence and categories (the self is to be efficiently managed through making a habit of: temperance, silence, order, resolution, frugality, industry, sincerity, etc. etc.). Franklin would have loved a chart for doing eye exercises in which one ticks off each five minute exercise/drill accomplished. Spontaneity and unexpected flashes of whimsy, clarity, and insight are scheduled out of this programmed propriety.
4. Franklin and others' ideals of order and regimentation ruled the formation of (eventually) compulsory public schooling. Benjamin Rush, father of American psychology and psychiatry, thought schooling was to be an advanced social therapy which would concern itself with the moulding of good citizens devoted to punctuality, discipline and order through memorized drills governed by the clock.
5. Americans by the 1700s had developed high repute as makers of clocks and locks. The first enclosed physical spaces. The second holds us to the concept of linear time.

Professor Welch says, 'We can appreciate the utter logic, so appropriate to be almost archetypal of the selling of glasses and timepieces together. All through the 19th century, in fact, glasses were promoted as the means to 'efficient vision' — the advertisements and lectures repeat the phrase constantly. These are tangible effects of a deep seated philosophy of life that created and sustained the

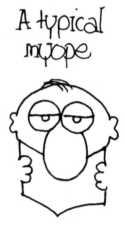

A typical myope

institutions and artifacts, the industry and habits that harnessed and organized the spontaneous and intuitive.'

There has however been a shift from mechanized industrial society to the service society of today where the employed are mainly involved with the collection, procession and transmission of information. And even this phase is rapidly on its way out. Economist Hazel Henderson realizes that the proliferation of the microchip computer will eventually eliminate the need for humans to be efficient extensions of machines where the body and mind are sacrificed to the goal.

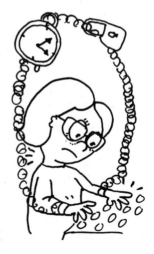

In her book, *Alternative Futures*, she proposes that that 'the micro processor has finally repealed the labour theory of value; there is really no possibility now of maintaining the fiction that human beings can be paid in terms of their labour'. Once the fear of having one's livelihood taken over by R2D2 has passed we might rejoice in the notion that the future holds great opportunity for personal growth. In the words of Australian Minister for Science and Welfare, Barry Jones in *Sleepers, Wake*, the future 'could be a golden age of leisure and personal development based on the cooperative use of resources'. I daresay this might include human as well as material resources.

A VIEW FROM THE PSYCHE

I find that discussion of a psychological genesis of myopia offers us the broadest vantage point of all because it can encompass all of the factors mentioned already. Emotions and our personalities are reflected in our diet, posture, work habits, repetition of family characteristics, even genetic predilections. It has been the myopic psychologists who with their penchant for peering into mental and emotional causes have occasionally been motivated by their own dull vision to ask the question, 'What do I and other myopes have in common besides our elongated eyeballs?' The studies that have been completed in the past few years have evolved a personality profile, a character for 'myopes'. This is not to deny that you may not be a variation on the theme. We discuss the stereotype here to help understand ourselves better and possibly come up with some home-grown solutions for change. Statistically astute psychological studies have shown that the typical myope:

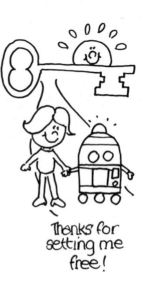

Thanks for setting me free!

1. Engages in near sector activities.
    (Do you love to read, stay at home, sit tight, keep in close?)
2. Is thin-skinned.
    (Do you feel hurt when someone yells at you? Are you the mouse or the doormat? Are you adept at nursing old wounds?)
3. Is proficient at academics, and has index file memory. (Did you get As on your exams and forget it all a month later?

Transforming the Myopic Character

Do you make lists in your mind and feel insecure if you don't know exactly what will be asked on the test?)

4.   Lives in a state of compressed anxiety and unconscious apprehension. (Do you ask yourself, 'Am I in the right place at the right time? What if I make a mistake?')

From behavioural optometry, we learn some other interesting perspectives about myopes. We find myopes have:

1.   Reduced peripheral awareness.
(Do you ever feel like you are walled in? Do you feel you have lost your basic connection to life's broader meaning?)
2.   A prolonged central fixation time.
(Do your eyes and mind tend to stick to things, repeatedly buzzing around the same topic. Do you get tired of this?)

From Reichian therapists, we observe that myopes:

1.   Move through space with chronically stiff shoulders and neck, frozen in a flinching posture.
(Do you carry your burdens on your shoulders? Are you preparing to be rejected?)
2.   Have limited eye contact.
(Do you look away when things get 'hot'? Do you cut off your feelings in your eyes?)

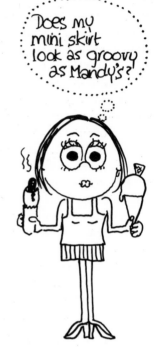

A few experiments have been done attempting to induce knotted-up myopes to relax enough to demonstrate a change in visual acuity under objective test conditions. In 1983, Wolfgang Gillessen presented a paper for an international conference on myopia concerned with imagery training involving forty-eight myopic patients of ophthalmologist Wolfgang Schultz-Zehden in Berlin. Results showed an improvement in attitude, 'A more relaxed passive attention was helpful for vision training exercises because the participants seemed to understand better what a less intensive, more passive looking style could be and how to maintain it through daily life'. The researchers found no change in acuity yet postulated that the instructor's reporting methods, few controls, and very little experimentation indicate that professional interests ought to take another look as, 'Reports of possible diagnostic benefits cannot be easily ignored [any longer]'.

In 1962, psychologist Charles Kelly did Ph.D. research on myopia. His paper demonstrated an objective change in myopic acuity ranging from 0.3 to 1.5 diopters after a classic Bates Method session. This study was published in an optometric journal and subsequently ignored.

The fact that a myope is often able to see better without glasses, but not exhibit a measureable change in axial length to an eye doctor doesn't obviate the fact that the brain is somehow not 'inter-

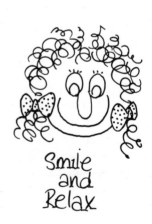

Smile
and
Relax

preting the blur better' but is actually rearranging the incoming data into a mentally clear image through hemispherical integration and the awesome powers of the imagination. In one case subject, acuity rose from 20/800 to 20/60. Are these people really seeing better, or is it just their imagination?

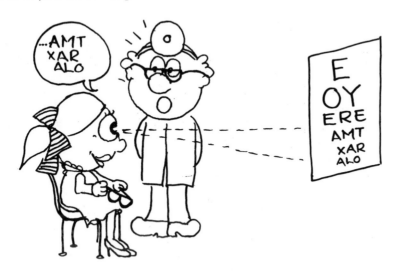

In 1977 a teacher of natural vision improvement did her Masters Degree thesis in psychology at UCLA using twelve of my myopic students as subjects. The results of her study are shown in chapter 17. The optometrist who performed the actual testing did not want his name mentioned.

I suspect that more and more research will emerge from psychologists concerning the mental aspects of myopia. Whether these studies will be read by the majority of physicians, optometrists and ophthalmologists is a moot point.

Let us range deeper into the fields of alternative psychology, the area I became so familiar with in 1967 in Southern California. An area that meant life to me.

VISION AND THE ENERGY STREAM

Therapists involved with the concepts of energy being 'blocked' or held back in the body observe the connection between eye disturbances and the ability to express the variety of human emotions. The fixed stare that accompanies refractive error is seen as a shrinking doorway that limits the *range* of sexual, visceral, and heart feelings that are communicated through the eyes. At a lecture given by bioenergetics therapist Alexander Lowen, he speaks of understanding the expression of feeling in the eyes as 'the energy pulsation between the head and the tail of the body ... that extends upward and downward from its center in the region of the solar plexus. It extends through the eyes above and into and through the genitals and legs below'. In Reichian terms, energy also means excitation, a 'charge' of energy that appears through the eyes resulting in a 'glow' or 'shine'. People with glowing eyes are assumed to have a strong sexual charge as well. At this point, I remember the fact that most female myopes develop blurred vision at age thirteen, when the hormonal flows and self-image of womanhood become entangled with the distorted images of sexuality and the role of women that can come through a sex-repressive culture.

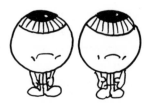

A fixed stare limits the range of sexual, visceral, and heart feelings...

If positive sexuality is something to be feared or embarrassed about then we will pull back our natural excitation from the eyes through a tightening of the muscles that are responding to emotional control via the autonomic nervous system. Lowen says, 'The person who suffers from myopia also has trouble in making eye contact and in expressing feelings through his/her eyes. I believe that the emotional disturbance is primary ... the visual disturbance develops secondarily as a result of strain.'

The Bioenergetic, Reichian, Neo-Reichian, and Rebirthing therapies that can bring back feeling into the eyes begin with raising one's energy level through fuller and deeper respiration. Fuller breathing heightens life energy flow and is sometimes followed by muscular relaxation, verbalizing, sounding, and eventually emotional resolution of the dammed-up feelings.

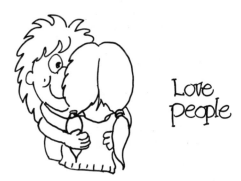

Love people

These kinds of therapies can be extremely helpful in cracking open one's armoring or shell if they are available to you. They are not a prerequisite. I've seen many myopic students improve their sight who've not had access to any therapies as such. The universe is replete with life energy. You will connect to it in your own ways.

HOW TO BE A PERFECT MYOPE

The culture, the educational process, family influences and our own unique wills and ways have come together to produce the person we are at this moment. Here we sit, wondering how it might be possible to change certain aspects of ourself, to pick up the reins of our lives more deliberately and move this whole show in another direction. To do so, let's examine and recognize the character that we have created so substantially. Then we'll look at ways to change our role while not taking anything personally. Here is the recipe for a total myopic character:

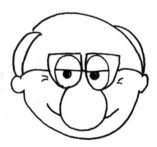

in the physical: Have an eyeball or two wherein the focal point of the entering light falls inside the eye. Develop tight jaws, neck and shoulders, hold the breath in, tummy tight. Ingest lots of flesh proteins and sugar.

in the emotions: Feel isolated. Feel incompetent but do compete. Prove to the world that you are worthy, for others just might basically disapprove of you. Bury all this.

in the mental: Think more than you imagine. Fantasize more than you create. Run through lines, scripts again and again in your head. Be unspontaneous in humor. Compare yourself to others unfavorably. Avoid making mistakes with a vengeance.

There are variations of the theme in America. The New York style myope is aggressive to cover the fear. The West Coast myope covers his/her anxiety with being spaced-out. There is the sweet country myope, the professional myope (the professor just after the facts), the artiste myope (jokes and hilarity cover insecurity), the homebody myope (shy and retiring, likes it that way), the bootstrap myope (those of us who grit our teeth even more and make sure we are not like any of the above).

Let us realize that our personality expressions are a momentary version of our inner essence, or our life energy, which is positive, pure and good. Personality is subject to labelling, to being put in a box, psychoanalyzed. You are in reality not to be labelled. You are not even a 'myope'. It is through the creative healing and balancing energy that comes from our core that we are able to change our characters, behaviors, and physical aspects. When this occurs, the labels no longer stick.

Reich used the analogy of an onion when speaking of human armoring (defence). The layers peel off in the process of therapy. Let's change the tearful, fearful awkward onion into a lotus. The myopic personality might look like the image on the next page. As you transform some of the mental/emotional factors underlying the glasses and the myopic behavior, you will bloom.

Myopia is an opportunity. Ride with the emotional ups and downs that release the creative emotional energy and lovingness that are tied up in your old habits. Use chart 2 as a springboard for mental thought pattern changes.

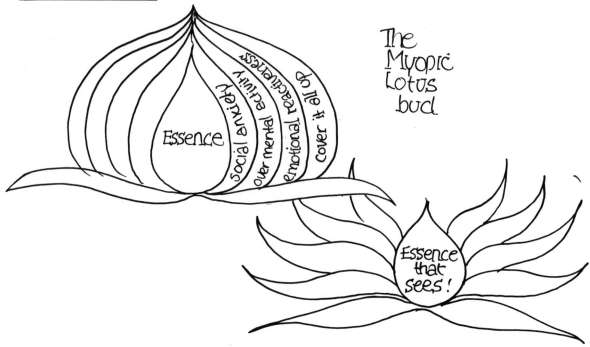

The Myopic Lotus bud

Essence

Social anxiety
Over mental activity
Emotional reactiveness
Cover it all up

Essence that sees!

Chart 2: **REWRITING THE SCRIPT**

	NEGATIVE	POSITIVE
Other people:	Everyone will think I am crazy.	I did it and everyone else joined in.
Physical danger:	Well, I didn't hit anybody.	I feel confident about driving.
'Missing out':	I feel so bad I wasn't there.	My cup of experience is always full and overflowing.
Perfectionism:	If I make a mistake, something disastrous will happen. (I will be unloved, rejected)	What's a mistake? I learn as I go along.
Paranoia:	People will ignore, dislike, or look at me with disdain or distaste.	I am radiantly beautiful. Other people love me.
Suppression:	I didn't say anything because I didn't want to hurt feelings.	I am able to express myself fully and lovingly to others.
Delayed Reactions:	I was so angry and upset I couldn't think of anything to say until a week later.	My mind is responsive and articulate.
Double split:	I know what to eat but I still eat junk.	All parts of my being join together in growing, improving, living.

Work through these issues with creativity and a sense of humor. When in a rut, ask for help from a therapist, a lover, a guide, a friend, yourself. A reluctance to ask for help often shows you believe you are less than perfect or not 'up to snuff', not worth the bother. We know better, don't we?

It doesn't matter which came first, the personality characteristics or the myopia. Look at yourself lovingly. Become aware. Whatever the reasons, in the course of things, your insight into self grows. The causative factors may then become known to you. Examples might be specific memories, or incidents that you will be able to relive and revise rather than repress.

Move. Move your eyes by doing the swings (See chapter 6). Move your mind, let go. Let go of the old stuff mentally and physically. Bring in the new:

'I am in a new world right at this moment.'

'I am in the midst of renewal and rebirth.'

'People adore me.'

'I am a beloved child of the universe.'

'Everything I thought was an error was an integral part of my learning to be me.'

'Wherever I am is perfect, appropriate, significant.'

'I am expanding my circle of energy and move with grace into the universe.'

'I am ready for the creativity of my intuitive mind/self to emerge and blend with my intellect.'

'I have the cosmic good person seal of approval.'

'I am a clear seer of distant beauties.'

Let go of your emotions through movement: breathing, running, yoga, dancing, laughing, yawning, all will stir up and stimulate your natural high spirits. Drop the ball a few times. Tell some jokes. Act out your naturally funny entertaining self with humorous stories. Reveal your hidden fears through storytelling and anecdotes. It is really ridiculous and funny to be repressed. It is painful too. Let the laughter and the tears of relief emerge together. Be less of an expert. Be a beginner. Do art, drawing from the child within you. Accept the burgeoning avid parts of yourself no matter what your age. Your active left brain would love to learn something new. Dive into unknown waters experiencing your fears as they slide out and away from you. Expand your action skills and you will be proud of yourself in a deeply satisfying way.

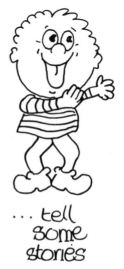

... tell some stories

Transforming the Myopic Character

Myopic people are extremely sensitive to their environments and to other people's thoughts, auras, gestures, and opinions. Otherwise, why would they need so much protection? This almost psychic receptivity that is usually naive and uneducated, gets masked by the defensive accoutrements of armoring, self put-downs, excess verbalizing, a numbed ability to love unconditionally. The softness is underneath all this. When you take off your compensating glasses, you will begin once more to open to the input from your environment, internally and externally.

It is possible to protect yourself in a way that will not interefere with your seeing. As a friend recently said to me when I was feeling anxious about some threatening psychic images I was seeing, 'Love is always your best protection'. This thought immediately calmed me and I was able to look at, learn from and transform the images without denying or ignoring them.

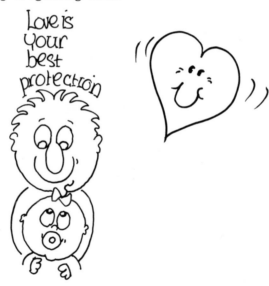

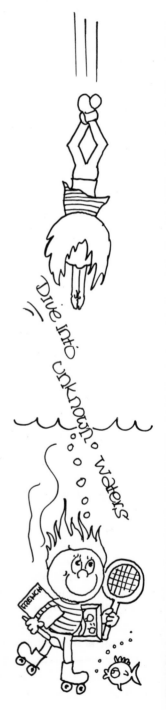

Myopes may carry emotional scars from the past due to their original tenderness. A gentle loving way of cleansing the past without hostile reactiveness is to use:

THE SOAP BUBBLE

Visualize yourself in the centre of an iridescent lustrous soap bubble whose surface deflects all darts and inadverdent slights. The image carrying light of inner and outer vision flows freely through your bubble. Now imagine a past event in which you felt drained or injured in some way. Call back to your bubble all the energy that you allowed to escape through that hole in your energy field. See the energy returning to you in colored streamers of light. Unrequited love, stepped on toes, callous primary teachers, slurs, misunder-

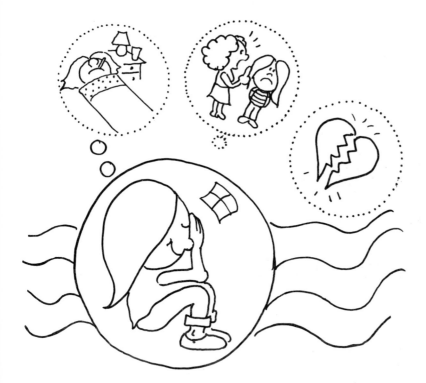

standings: their aches all flow away, their scars dissolve as you reestablish you high level center in relation to the wholeness of life around you. No longer is there a need to shut out any part of your experience — past present or future — as you perceive the lushness of physical reality in serene clarity.

Chapter 3

Transforming Hyperopia, Astigmatism and Sexuality

You might say, 'Janet, I am not a myope and some of the things you talked about in the last chapter apply to me too.' This is true, because none of us are really confined to labelled boxes. Sometimes we're one way and sometimes another. Sometimes we are left brain robots, sometimes right brain space cases. Perhaps we are echoing the fact that our visual system naturally moves from myopia to hyperopia. We reach out and we pull back in. Homeostasis brings us back to a mobile centre of mind, body and eyesight. It is getting stuck at one point or another that freezes us as myopic, hyperopic or astigmatic.

HYPOTHESES ABOUT HYPEROPES

This area has been talked about less than myopia. It is no less important. Observations from friends and clients who wore thick magnifiers, often from early childhood, is that a basic repression of energy expression is happening in them as well as in myopes. It simply is manifested in the visual system as a foreshortening of the eyes. In hyperopia the focal point of the light entering the eye falls behind the retina rather than in front as in myopia. This is often accompanied in early years by squint, temper tantrums, a sudden wildness that contrasts with the myopes' sedateness (who are trying to be so good). The hyperopes often become dyslexic in school scrambling letters and numbers while the myopes take all the first grade accolades. What's happening with the hyperopes?

Charles Kelly, from his Neo-Reichian perspective on hyperopes, feels that hyperopes hold back anger at their first level of repres-

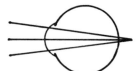

A Hyperopic eye

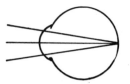

A normal eye

sion. My observation of hyperopes is that they are as over-controlled as myopes, but they are meeting authority with authority, rather than with fear. Hyperopes like to turn into the officials, to make sure things are done right. These can be myopic characteristics also. However, the hyperope's motives come not so much from wanting approval from others as from a hunger for reassurance from the self.

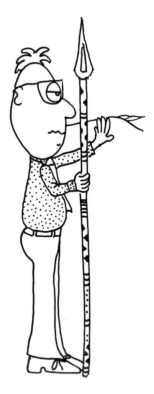

The hyperopic visual posture is steely, almost warlike. They are the sentinels of the visual world. They are able to detect the distant approach of the enemy across the plain. They act sure of themselves. Their eyes often look piercing. Their necks are erect and boardlike. Their chest is often frozen and bony. They can get righteously vehement about things. Often the hypers, who are actually seeing from the picture-giving right hemisphere, are most sure of themselves in the overseeing areas of business — public relations, stock broking. When they screw their eyes down to the pre-requisite paperwork in these fields they end up in thick bifocals, trifocals, etc. with fists full of irritating glasses. Personal relationships are fine but let someone step in too close to the heart and eyes, and the hyper backs off. Those red-hot feelings might get touched off.

IN A WORLD THAT'S TOO BIG

In the beginning, near things are unmanageable and too close for comfort without your glasses. The plus lenses prescribed for hypers allow that discomfort to remain internally and hold you in the thrall of artificial magnification. They make the world huge, sending it even farther away metaphorically speaking. When people look at your face your eyes will be magnified to them (It's Little Riding Hood, to the wolf, 'My what big eyes you have'.) It will take even more effort to turn your attention to the close and small things in life. In the distance, without glasses, you are probably using both hemispheres. When you look at the printed page, the left hemisphere which takes care of details and specifics, turns off. There is massive blur for reading — pain, discomfort and anxiety about accomplishing those technical tasks that you direct so well. Without the glasses the hypers whose ability to perform left-brain specific tasks appears completely dependent on the existence of magnification, panic. 'I can't think (or hear) without my glasses', said Valerie who at fifty-four had been wearing plus lenses since childhood. The hyperopes who are unable to entertain and express their angry frustration drop down into fear, suspicion and self-doubt.

PEACEMAKING

Consider using the following thoughts to ease both conscious and unconscious mental habits.

'I am approachable.'

'I am receptive to the little things in life.'

'My energy moves out into the world clearly and peacefully.'

'I express myself to others beneficially and gracefully.'

'Anger is what I move through and it moves through me.'

'My eyes are softly receiving the words and details of the close worlds, the inner worlds.'

'I am able to be creatively rational.'

'My trust in others and myself is complete.'

'The world is taking care of itself.'

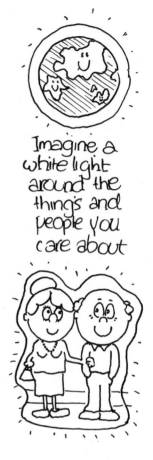

Imagine a white light around the things and people you care about

Visualize a white light around the earth. This light streams from you or from any point you choose. Its essence is loving clarity. Imagine the light flowing around specific people and situations in your more immediate range. A self-sufficient and self-balancing force permeates your friends, relatives and neighbors as you relax your vigilance in favor of the white light flowing from your imagination. The world is taking care of itself, leaving you free to develop. Go for your own creative urges — a stroll in the garden perhaps; a white butterfly may alight on your sleeve. You will see it clearly. Mentally make peace with the world in small ways. Rather than running the campaign, I suggest sitting with a flower or a cloud or a small person. Play with balls — tennis, ping-pong, squash, a simple game of catch. Loosen up and enjoy yourself in small ways as you absorb the principles that will release you from glasses.

IS THERE AN ASTIGMATIC CHARACTER?

Physically astigmatism is a warp across the cornea (less often across the lens) causing a sensation akin to looking through old glass. Lower degrees of it come and go through the day. Many times it is related to simple eyestrain. People tell me they had glasses for astigmatism during their college years and never needed them again afterwards. When emotional and mental tension lifts, mild astigmatic conditions disappear.

Astigmatic distortion can be found by itself or in conjuction with myopia, hyperopia, even presbyopia. Higher degrees of it become locked in place by corrective lenses and possibly by corresponding mind/body character adaptations.

Consider with me: what actually is our experience with astigmatism? The eyes smart and burn. They fatigue quickly. Straight lines repeat themselves, the moon multiplies.

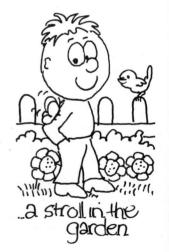

...a stroll in the garden

If astigmatic eyes could speak, they might say, 'Ouch, the visual world is hurting me!' and 'What I see is painful and exhausting.' You might, at some time, question the origins of such feelings. Also, think about which eye carries the astigmatism. In the philosophy of iridology the right eye represents the left-brain and the left eye the right-brain. I speculate that the astigmatic stress I had in my right eye related to my childhood resistance to the mundane outer world. I retreated into fairytales and books to avoid interacting with the 'pain and confusion' of the real world.

Many people, including Robert Mendelsohn, author of *Confessions of a Medical Heretic*, have suggested that the high incidence of astigmatism in babies and children could be a response to birth trauma, including forcep deliveries, glaring hospital lights, and the common American practice of automatically placing preventive caustic solutions in the eyes of new born babies.

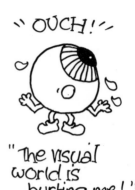

RELEASING THE PAIN

By extrapolating from my own past experience with astigmatism and from talking with students, some thoughts emerge that may be helpful.

'My visual world is coherent and smooth.'

'The world is honest with me. It talks straight with me.'

'My eyes receive lines and shapes passively, peacefully.'

'I know what's required of me in the big world — to love and to be myself.'

'The world is soft, gentle and receptive to me.'

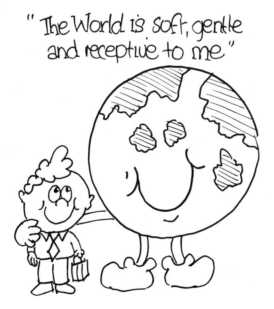

A REBIRTHING IMAGE

Close your eyes and visualize with these thoughts. 'I am here. I feel my graceful harmonious body moving fluently from enclosing darkness into spreading light. The hands of the light are soft, warm and gentle. They hold me and assure me as I sense my physical boundaries sliding into the curving, coherent, pulsing body that is my perceiving self. Humming sounds fall into my ears like trickling water. I want to open my eyes because I shall be delighted, welcomed by love-shiny faces, by twinkling colors that will weave a lifelong fascinating amusement for me.'

If you even minimally reactivate your eyes through the animating activities described above (and later), it is possible you will experience some emotional ups and downs. Emotion is energy in motion. Pure emotion is energy undifferentiated. You could call an emotional feeling 'happiness', 'anger', 'fear', 'grief', 'frustration', 'joy'. The extension power of your emotion is the reach of your spirit. How 'emotional' you can be is not how much pathos you can conjure or how much you choose to hang around with negative feelings, but how strongly you feel about life. A flexible, emotional (spirited) person who experiences fully the ebb and flow of both positive and negative aspects of life returns to a joyful centre.

The physical and mental movements of the natural vision activities open and clear a channel through your body/mind. Meaningful experiences will then happen through your eyes.

Be generous with the ups and downs of your vision. Also be not surprised by fluctuations in motivation. This is natural. It is the desire to see clearly that carries you through periods of discouragement or indifference.

SEEING SEXUALITY

Sexual actions and interests are generated by the movement of universal creative energy. If this energy is blocked in us our sexual expressions will become distorted rather than enjoyed. Many of us struggle with the low vibrational depictions of sexuality that come through the mass media. There is no doubt that the sexual energy is called forth by visual images outwardly and inwardly. Through our own pleasurable and positive experiences of sexuality that involves our total being — from body to mind to imagination to spirit — we are eventually able to live within and through a healthy life-expansive sexual universe.

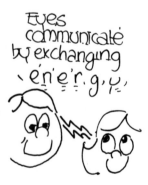
Eyes communicate by exchanging energy

The eyes are superb transmitters of strong clear messages that would be enfeebled by the use of words alone. Eyes comment and communicate by exchanging energy.

The primary sexual eye contact is that between mother and baby. The erotic sensations of breast-feeding wrapped in tenderness and caring foster the eventual communication between lovers. A high voltage beam from eyes to eyes opens up a process of healing, fusing, playing — the shared expression of one's precious life content.

Sharing the depth of vision possible through another's eyes creates an intensification of the light vibrations. A seeing quality is engendered that goes beyond the ordinary. It has the flavor of the 'ultra visual' flashes of clarity that bring natural vision students into class brimming with enthusiasm about their sight.

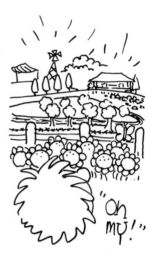

The same flexibility, receptivity and flowingness that catalyzes clear vision also promotes positive sensual and sexual events. Women have spoken with me about the fact that they get headaches during sexual contact. When looking at the situation we find that several thing are going on during that opportunity.

1. The eyes are tightly closed while the mind is thinking: 'I should be feeling X or Y.' 'Why aren't I responding?' 'Am I doing this right?' The left brain ego is running pre-programmed tapes.
2. The back of the neck is tight, shutting off the sexual flow up into the eyes. The teeth are clenched.
3. Your body is there, the mind is thinking about making dinner. Is this sexual boredom? Is there an inkling of guilt about this?

RELAX AND GLOW

Open your eyes, see where you are. Roll your head from side to side (a few snuggly kisses on tight neck muscles are good). Open your mouth and sound airy sighs. Turn your mind to images rather than thoughts by knowing that —

1. You are energy caring for energy.
2. You are being yourself and that's enough.
3. The sexual energy will rise into your visual system creating a kaleidoscope of brilliant colors and moving images that will carry your whole being into the place you want to go.

THE RED IN THE GREEN

The sexual energy is traditionally and spiritually carried by the color red. You might use this color in visualizations to prepare your physical system for the current of vital energy that moves through us as we evolve into aliveness. Then when we are alone with wholeness our seeing will embrace the sexual energy expressed by nature in the flowers, trees, the magical rainbow — imbibing the beauties of the physical world at every turn. An example is the following personal story of significant perception through sexual energy sharing.

While embracing my companion, I looked up into the blue and white dappled sky. In that moment a sparkling stream of energy sprang up through my heart and out the top of my head. My thinking mind was captivated by the change in perception. I was seeing the lush green grass as if I were the grass. Something in the centre of me cleared with the depth, emerald emotion and pure exuberance of rich growing grass. I closed my eyes and was greeted by the same blades of grass blazoning forth in crimson red. At their roots I could see a deeper orange-red. Lifting my attention to the space above the grass I saw living flames licking the air and, astonished, I opened my eyes and still saw the red in the green. I realized the significance of seeing red with green could be dissolved in a scientific statement about retinal chemistry, yet I was seeing them simultaneously with my eyes open. The scientist part of me was willingly tugged off into the art gallery memory of impressionistic painters. A layer of understanding settled around my mind. Cezanne and other impressionists had used complementary colors side by side to create a visual illusion of aliveness and light in nature. There was another bunch of sexually-interested originators who were at first derided and then beloved.

The red glow lasted for a long time in my eyes. Grace filled me up and flavored the tears that dripped off my cheeks. I poured these unspoken feelings into the eyes of my friend.

Chapter 4

The Return of Clarity

We move now to set the foundation for backing you out of glasses. You may have to use your current spectacles to read this next section. This is understandable. Read it first then put the book down and go through the activities as best you are able without glasses. Another idea is to read the instructions into a tape recorder and play them back to yourself.

MAKING FRIENDS WITH THE BLUR

Sit in a comfortable position and place your middle fingertips gently on the prominences of your forehead. Run the following thoughts through your mind: 'I do not *have to* see anything clearly. I appreciate the vision that I am expressing right now. I cease fighting with the blur, cease resenting it. I realize that this is my actual vision and I accept it. In fact I enjoy the blur. I am able to get around in familiar spaces. I am able to breathe deeply. I may not recognize my friends across the street or be able to see the addresses in the phone book, but this is temporary. I am able to relax and let go in this watercolor world. I shall acquire an understanding of how I created this world. And how I will transform it into clarity.'

Allow yourself to perceive and appreciate the way the visual world appears. Take some time for this. Breathe deeply and yawn as you would in a well-known chair with old familiar companions. Yawn fully. Several times. Stretching out your arms.

Acknowledge yourself as the decision maker in your life. The eyesight you are experiencing right now is yours, totally acceptable and appropriate for this moment. You accept the present state and know that you are able to change it through your active participation in the life energy itself.

Take a deep breath. Feel your mind soften. Still holding your forehead, continue with these kinds of thoughts: 'I know that the world around me is alive and always changing. My eyes, my mind, are also mobile and vital, vibrant. I am flexible and I am willing to embark on this adventure of self-healing. Nature and the wonderful resources of my creative mind are supporting me.'

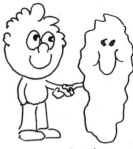

Make friends with the blur

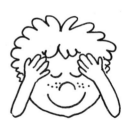

YAWNING IS GOOD

Ah, those yawns. We restrict energy flow through our whole being by unconsciously holding our breath. A bit of relaxed yawning opens the door to fuller breathing. When giant yawns begin to emerge, you may notice a change, a brightening, a depth in the world around you. Pause and appreciate. You have relaxed and become more receptive, more attuned to the space in which you are living.

Imagine you are a tawny golden lion lounging in the warm sun of an African plain. Your friends and family are draped over tree branches, slumbering. They're playing languidly in the afternoon shimmer in the soft belly of the toasty earth. You stretch your forepaws forward, open your great mouth wide and yawn hugely exhaling with a gentle roar.

That felt so good you do it again. This time you contract your sinuous shoulders. Tighten them upward and forward as you inhale. They release down into feline suppleness as you exhale. Sound flows out of your open throat in a full leonine purr.

The 'impolite' YAWN: Humans control their expression by controlling their breathing. The yawn is the most naturally freeing and the fullest kind of breathing possible when we have a spontaneous need for fresh oxygen, stretching of muscles, and a change of pace. Yet we have been taught to suppress yawning. Let us change this state of affairs.

Yawning opens the jaw hinge and sets the masseter muscle free. This jaw muscle tightens with too much thinking and grinds the teeth through the night. Another muscle called the temporalis assists the masseter in closing the jaw. Since it attaches along the sides of the head and in the area of the temple, tension in this muscle can cause headaches. When the masseter and temporalis are tight, the muscles around the mouth, in the cheeks and around the eyes also tighten up. A few good yawns will contract and relax all these muscles together. Your teeth, jaw, brain, and eyes will thank you.

Unconscious messages pass between people all the time. Sometimes these undercurrents of communication are more important than the rationalities that come out of the mouth. One person yawns and others follow without thinking about it. Carry it even further. Have occasional yawning parties with children and friends. Everyone will enjoy themselves once they get over their inhibitions, tummies soften, annoying thoughts are released, cleansing tears run down the cheeks, indeed there are so many benefits to unbridled yawning I want to list them for you:

1. Yawning brings fresh oxygen into body cells including the eyes and brain.
2. Yawning contracts then releases the muscles related to the eyes. A really good yawn will contract and expand muscles

The giant yawn will emerge...

YAWNNN

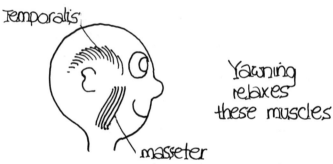

from the top of your head to the tips of your toes — including the shoulder or trapezius muscles, the eyes (orbicularis oculi), the neck (neck flexors), the belly (the abdominals and solar plexus area).

3. Yawning is capable of changing emotional states from negative to positive.
4. Yawning changes the pH of the blood reducing toxicity levels in your whole system.
5. It opens the mind to new experiences.
6. Yawning helps to detoxify the liver and to balance the energy in the liver meridian.
7. It wakes you up in the morning. It calms you down for deep restful sleep at night.
8. Yawning stimulates the production of refreshing tears that bathe naturally tired eyes and moisten chronically dry eyes.
9. It relaxes the solar plexus area and tummy muscles that accompany indigestion. Well-being comes into your midriff.
10. Write down what yawning does for you.

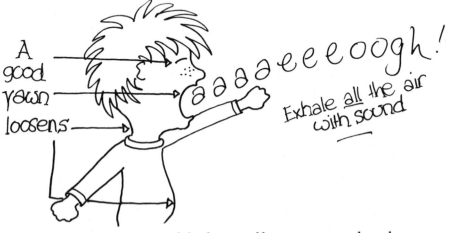

If you want to yawn and find yourself amongst people, who have not yet rid themselves of the yawn prejudice, simply excuse yourself and say 'I am so relaxed in your company, I just start to yawn.' Likely the other person will smile and join you.

SOUND YAWNING

Once past a certain age, we no longer make sounds. However, no decent yawn would be caught without its sound. Making a sound requires that the mouth open (yes, fully open). Show your teeth, tongue and throat to the world as you inhale, then exhale through the mouth with gusto. Do this with your own unique roar, croon, aria, shriek, or lament. Whatever your sound, let it come out uncensored. You will get used to hearing yourself relax. Gradually your family and friends will get used to it. They may even chime in.

It is completely natural to exhale with sound when you yawn. We are instruments of sound. However most people have been silenced from childhood except for rational (left-brain) speech. Humming, crooning, burbling, squealing, groaning, trilling and singing have been quietened. Throats get tight, jaws sit in tension and grinding of the teeth occurs. Self-consciousness and embarrassment imprison effectively any non-verbal spontaneous sound. Let's change this.

It takes energy to inhibit natural human expressions including a sometimes spontaneous urge to sigh, growl, or exult. Reopening to any extent the pre-verbal expressions of your voice will help to release energy and relax your body and mind. Sound itself when combined with imagery becomes an effective, inwardly joyous way to energize the visual system.

1. Sound carries negative emotions, thoughts and vibrations away from your centre.
2. Sound itself becomes a positive emotion (energy in motion) which you generate yourself.
3. Rhythmic humming stimulates the creative seeing (right) brain.
4. Sound physically vibrates, loosens, reenergizes nerve, muscle tissue, and bones in the body. It 'microadjusts' the bones of the head surrounding the eyes and optic nerve.
5. You are able to regulate the sound, its timbre, tone, volume and direction. You are able to send healing vibrations to any part of your self with sound.

TUNING YOUR HARMONIUM

Sit with your eyes closed comfortably. Exhale every scrap of old stale air from your lungs. Open your mouth and inhale into your tummy and chest. Exhale with a HUMMMMMMMMM, getting all the air out. Continue humming for a while, exploring the ups and downs and vibratory potential of your HUMMMMMMMMM. Locate a pitch that feels vibratory. Notice where you feel the vibration in your body. Intensify the HUMMMMMMMMM. Put more breath power behind it until you have a warm round solid sound.

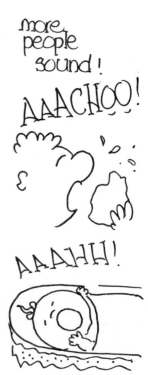

LESS MACHINE SOUND

RRRMMMM...

BANG BANG!

more people sound!

AAACHOO!

AAAHH!

Open your mouth and let the sound stream out. Imagine sending this sound into your hands. Do this until your hands glow and thrum gently. Send the sound into your left eye. Its pitch may rise as you move it higher in your body. You may feel your cheekbones vibrate first, then the sinus cavities and the nose. Send the gentle but strong HUMMMM into your right eye. Imagine the sound waves moving through eyelids, eye muscles, optic nerves, eye tissue, blood vessels.

Imagine that your HUMMMMMMMMMMing sound is now flowing forth from each of your eyes and is meeting at a point directly in front of you. Eyes are still closed. Visualize this point lighting up and glowing with a color you choose. Do this for five more breaths and then allow your eyes to open.

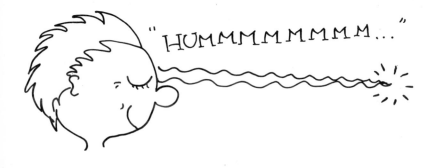

Imagine that your Humming sound is flowing from your eyes and meeting at a point directly in front of you...

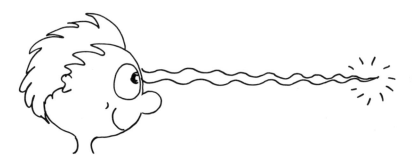

Allow your eyes to open.

RESOUNDING COLOR

To broaden your ability to imagine color, combine it with sound. With eyes closed, ask for the sound of a particular color, e.g. emerald green, to come to you. Exhale fully, followed by a total inhalation. Open your mouth and let the sound radiate out of you. Whatever sound you get is it. No judgment of right or wrong in sound relationships, please. Exhale and sound with green several times. Then go to some other colors: daffodil yellow, sunset orange, heavenly blue, chinese dragon red, lustrous lavender, french violet, deep purple.

The Return of Clarity

LOOSENING UP WITH MASSAGE

Increasing your breathing capacity, your movement and your whole life expression will give you more energy. Sometimes this tide of energy rises up in you and runs into old holding patterns. Eyes may get tired. Shoulders may tighten up. Yawning and transforming thoughts will help with this. Yet when the going gets rough sometimes direct muscle massage is called for.

It is wonderful to have someone else massage you. Find recruits for this if possible. Yet when no one else is available it is 'do it yourself' time. Instead of suffering stoically with stiff aching muscles, take a hold and massage yourself.

The upper trapezius muscle (shoulder) inevitably gets tight when there is stress in the eyes (and ears as well). It tilts the chin and pulls on the shoulder blades. Take a hold of your left shoulder muscle with your right hand. 'Pick' the muscle up and hold it. You can also HUMMMM as you do this allowing the tension to escape through your voiced sound. Then knead the muscle like bread dough. End up by brushing it off briskly with your hand. The right shoulder deserves the same. Grasp it with your left hand. Supporting your elbow with the other hand may give you more leverage.

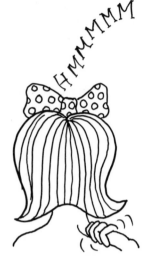

Knead the muscle like bread dough!

TUNING UP YOUR EARS

Eyes and ears are closely related. As babies, we turn our heads in the direction of tinkling bells, touch with our eyes, then reach out with our hands. Later on, loud discordant music, undesirable arguments, piercing sounds may cause us to 'switch off' our ears and hearing. To re-attune hearing, massage a circle around your ears. Follow this with a thorough massage of the ears themselves. This will turn the audio centres in your brain on again and give your ears and head a lovely warm expanded feeling.

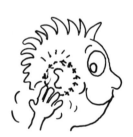

MIRRORING THE BEAUTY

As you remove your glasses and become a visual animating artist, your eyes begin to sparkle, friends make complimentary remarks, and your face changes.

Tight straining eyes locked behind glasses are always accompanied by tension in facial muscles that make us look older and tired, or worried, or suspicious. The three sets of muscle groups that follow the state of the eyes (and mind) are the Four Frowners, the Squinters, and the Washboard Forehead Makers. Each of these when contracted carries a clear communication with it.

For eighteen years, Paul Edman and Wallance Friesen, psychologists at the University of California, San Francisco, studied facial expression and body movement under the aegis of NIMH

(National Institute of Mental Health). Cross-cultural research revealed that universal facial expressions 'freeze' the emotions through the muscles of the face. The expression on your face always communicates your feelings to other people whether anyone, including you, is consciously aware of it. Even when saying 'OK.' to the question, 'How are you feeling?', your face reveals what kind of company your thoughts have been keeping. You may think that your face is blank, yet chronic tension in muscles belies your neutrality. Our 'frozen affect' faces may look sad (*the corners of the lips are turned down*) or suprised (*the brows are slightly raised*), angry (*the brows are lowered* or *the lips tightened*) or worried (*the brows are slightly raised and drawn together*). These unspoken facial communications display the chronic states of our minds, eyes, and emotions.

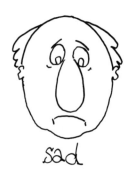

sad

There are several reasons why I feel it is important to be aware of and relieve the eye-related stress and tension in our faces which the wearing of glasses often aids in masking and maintaining:

1. We may be sending messages that are quite different from those we wish to convey to our friends and loved ones. For example, a mother who pinches her brow together with constant worry may not be aware that she is communicating disapproval to her child. 'I thought she was mad at me,' the child says. Squinting denotes sadness, anger or disgust. Happiness, on the other hand, draws up the corners of the mouth. The eyes sparkle and glisten, the forehead is smooth.
2. The facial tension sends an auto-feedback into your psyche which results in self-disdain.
3. The tight facial expressions help hold the eyes in a stare.
4. Unlocking facial muscles which hold unconscious negative emotions tends to rid one of those undesirable traits.
5. Relaxed faces look younger, are more attractive and SEE better.

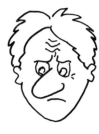

surprised

ERASING THE FROWNS, SQUINTS AND WASHBOARDS

People with visual blur who leave off glasses without utilizing mind/body relaxation often end up frowning and squinting. The presbyopes who stave off reading glasses and hyperopes who are pushing the printed world away, develop a washboard forehead by raising the frontalis muscle.

Look in the mirror. Who is that person and what is she/he saying? Smile at yourself then lie down or sit comfortably with a cushion under your elbows and do one or both of the following actions for smoothing away the frown:

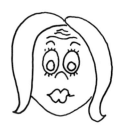

angry

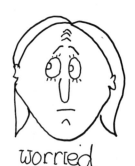

worried

The Return of Clarity

1. Frown and find the muscle with your fingertips that is acting out this concern. With your thumb and forefinger, pick up a tiny section of that muscle and pinch it together quickly, briefly. Feel the 'ouch'. Send a conscious command to your left brain along with the 'ouch' telling it to release this muscle. Then HUMMMMMM for three seconds to activate the right brain. The reason for this little procedure is to release the muscle cells from the trying, worrying, conscious left brain and put it back in the care of the relaxed, creative right brain. This is akin to a process used in 'Touch for Health' called the 'spindle cell technique'. Do this action all along the muscle responsible for unconscious habitual frowning.

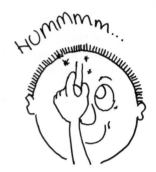

Use the spindle cell method

2. Place your fingertips on your brows and stretch them apart erasing the frown. Maintain this action and close your eyes. Imagine: 'In the center of my forehead is a tiny round jewel. Its center glows with an inner light that is beginning to radiate outward. The circumference of its glow is just a couple centimetres at first. The light is a shimmering lustrous lavender with iridescent streaks of pink and gold flashing at its perimeter. As I breathe the light expands. When this happens, the skin of my forehead smooths out and becomes broad and even. As the light spreads outward it chases away all impish, muddied, weighty concerns. My forehead expands, spreading in all directions until it is like a calm ocean.'

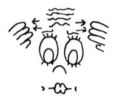

With your fingertips stretch your brows apart

3. Use the spindle cell method on the frontalis muscle. Its fibres run up and down so you'll be able to use your thumb and forefinger to pinch in little stitches up and down. Send the strong request to the left brain to release the muscle, then pause and HUMMMMM. Then massage thoroughly along your hairline where the frontalis inserts.

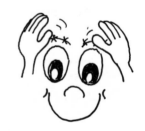

4. Place your fingertips just at the top of your eyebrows. Give a *very slight* downward pull and hold while you run these kinds of thoughts and images through your mind: 'My brows are two brave albatross who have flown a long and arduous journey across ocean. Now they have reached the end of their flight and are coming down to rest on a flat strand of warm sandy beach. Their great wings flow downward and rest snugly at their sides. The noble birds' heartbeats slow. They look forward to a long serene sojourn at the side of the gently lapping ocean. My eyebrows are these birds.'

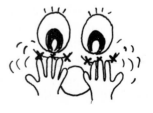

Close your eyes. Firmly and tenderly place your middle fingers on the edge of the bone beneath your eyes. Press and make a tiny circle for a few seconds. Move your fingers slightly and do the same. Move all around your eyes this way, shifting to the thumbs for the upper bone above your eyes.

Renewal of visual expression and perception accompanies relaxation of facial musculature. Soon, the attention and tension leaves your eyes and you feel as if you are seeing with your whole face. Eventually you will see with your whole body.

RELEASING THE BOTTLENECK

People with tight eyes generally have tight necks as well. The stiff-necked' person is maintaining his/her coping mechanisms by constant tension in the side neck flexors that turn the head from side to side, and in the back neck extensors which nod the head up and down and hold it erect against gravity. You have every right to release your own neck from an unconscious noose. In his book on restoring learning ability for children and adults, Paul Dennison says, 'If the neck is open, relaxed and loose, the body and mind can work together. When the neck is closed and tight, it actually becomes a valve to shut off energy.'

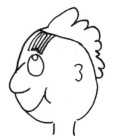

The frontalis muscle

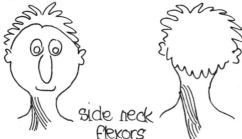

side neck flexors

Reach back with the middle fingers of each hand. Gently and firmly press into the base of your neck. Pull the muscles away from your spine. Lift your hands and move them to the area just above this. Again release the neck muscles to the side. Continue in this fashion right up to the base of your skull. Do it slowly, languidly, with rhythmic breathing. Imagine you're being massaged by the greatest physiotherapist in the world.

These up and down neck muscles attach to your weighty head at the base of the skull. Use your thumbs to press in the hollows you find there. Press for three deep breaths then move slightly to the sides and press again. Release that whole area extending from the corners of your mastoid bones to the center back point of your head.

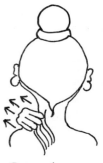

Pull the muscle away from the spine

FREEDOM OF EXPRESSION

Beside allowing energy to flow up your spine into the visual centers at the back of your head, soft neck muscles also signify an ability to say 'yes' to life. Activation of back neck extensors move our heads up and down for a non-verbal 'yes'. When it is appropriate to say 'no', the softened side neck muscles express that surety of 'no, that's enough' or 'no, that's not a helpful thing to do'. When people have repressed their 'no' ability, their resulting anger and sternness is held in those rigid side neck muscles.

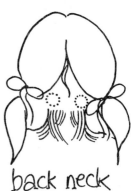

back neck extensors

The Return of Clarity

By doing the movement activities in this book that involve free motion of the head and neck you may develop a quicker 'hotline' from your body to your mind. Tensions previously unperceived will make themselves known, available for resolution and change.

THE KEY TO THE TREASURE

With our expanded definition of vision from chapter 1, you can set out with optimism to reexperience your 'lost' visual clarity. Self-balancing and self-healing means you use your own creative action and that you take complete responsibility for your state of well-being. We have said that vision is energy. More vision means more energy. This increase of energy will flow through you on all levels, physical, emotional, mental. This is the same as increasing your ability to experience pleasure. Wilhelm Reich told us about pleasure anxieties which arise when the positive life energy which has been held back begins to flow once more. The anxiety which increased energy sometimes activates can be experienced as lethargy, ennui, depression, scepticism, jitteryness, etc. These are temporary blocks to the irrepressible positive life energy that created both you and your vision in the first place. If you have decided that you basically desire to change your vision, but are lackadaisical about activating your knowledge, simply recognize that it is *pleasure* you are putting off.

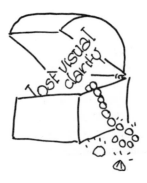

Chapter 5

Stepping Out of Glasses

If your vision is fairly blurred and you need glasses to meet the demands of your chosen lifestyle, it will be necessary to obtain a pair of 'transition glasses' that will give your eyes room to change and still allow you to drive and work safely and comfortably. 'Transition glasses' are lenses which are stepped down in curvature. Most eye doctors will have given you a correction in your glasses which allow you to read the 'normal' line of the chart. In America this is the '20/20' line. This means that from a distance of 20 feet you are able to read a letter of a certain height and a certain kind of typeface. This ability is subjective. You're mentally recognizing the letter and giving the right response. Optometrists and eye doctors also use an 'objective' way of determining the prescription for your glasses. They will look into the eye with a retinoscope. By optical means the retinoscope measures the refractive state of the eyes which is then compared with the subjective findings. The data obtained is then translated into a certain curvature which is ground into your glasses. This curvature is measured in diopters and is described on your prescription as a + or − numeral, (e.g. − 3.00 D for myopia and + 3.00 D for hyper and presbyopia).

DRIVING SAFELY

In most states in America the visual requirement for drivers is not 20/20 but 20/40. This means that the letter you have to correctly identify is one that a 'normal' sighted person is able to read at 40 feet. In countries where the metric system is used these numbers are 6/6 for correction to 'normal' vision; and 6/12 for reduced transition glasses.

There will come a time for people who are moving through stepped down glasses to have the restriction removed from their drivers' licences. I had my strong myopic and astigmatic correction reduced to 20/40 twice. I wore these weakened glasses for driving

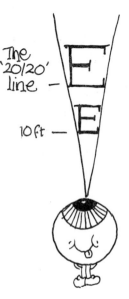

The '20/20' line —

10 ft —

until I realized that I could possibly pass the California driving vision test without lenses. This I did, as have many of my students over the past eighteen years. Some of these students went a couple of times to take the vision test. You can return *as often as you like* until the fact that you are taking a *test* (a vision turn-off in itself) no longer emotionally interferes with your relaxed sight.

SEEING IN THE DARK

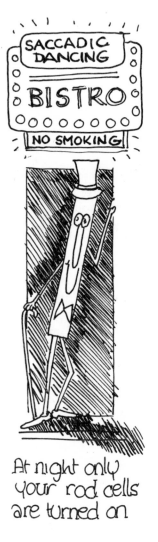

You may find that your visual capacity is lower at night than in the daytime. This is common. As your visual confidence grows and the movement games in the next chapters become more integrated into your life, your night vision will improve. In the meantime if you find you need to continue wearing reduced glasses for night-time driving, even after passing the driving test, do so until you can *confidently* discard glasses. It appears that night vision can lag behind daytime seeing for two reasons. First, the lowering light no longer stimulates the cone (color and detail receptor) cells that are active in daylight. In the dim light only your rod (light and shadow receptor) cells are turned on. We have no color and less detail at night.

The daylight receptive cone cells congregate more in a centralized part of your retina. The rod cells are scattered over the whole retina and are totally absent in the fovea centralis.

If you stare directly at something at night, your unstimulated cones will give you nothing but a blank spot in the center of your visual field. The best possible night vision comes from rod stimulation, which is strongly induced by the scanning and sketching which you'll learn in the next chapter.

At night only your rod cells are turned on

The second factor in night vision is circulation. The rod cells require an unhindered supply of oxygen to function at their best. Your scanning motions and deep breathing will help the rod cells get the fuel they need to sort out the lights and the shadows.

WHEN TO USE TRANSITION GLASSES

Transition (or T-) glasses are to be used for driving of course, in your work if needed, and perhaps in the back seat at the theater. Begin going without glasses at home, in your neighborhood, and where the environment is familiar. It is not a case of 'throw away your glasses'. It is a matter of weaning yourself from dependency upon them as soon and as comfortably as possible. Since seeing better is a matter of releasing tied-up energy, many of the activities found in this book are designed to help you take care of yourself while your whole brain and being are getting accustomed to the

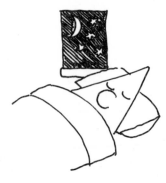

increased freedom of no glasses. Energy will flow as you loosen up your visual system.

If your blur is moderate or slight, you have no restriction that requires the wearing of corrective lenses on your drivers' licence, or you don't drive or work under pressure, leave off your glasses entirely. The optometric concept is that glasses compensate for eyestrain. Therefore *you* keep in mind that the games you are about to make a part of your life are designed to transform the *primary causes* of your blur and strain. If we are going to give your visual system a chance to rebalance itself, no glasses are in order.

Taking any kind of a test is an art. You are considered ignorant or incapable until you prove differently. It is a prime opportunity for many people to 'switch off' part of their brain and ability. The pressure and/or competition involved, often the attitude of the examiner, and the environment will directly affect your ability to respond in that moment. The lessons in relaxation and the Thrill of the Great White Glow (see chapter 14), plus attitude transformation, will help you in passing future eye tests. This applies to driving, piloting and career vision requirements.

REDUCING READING GLASSES

If you wear glasses only for close activity, it is also important to give your eyes room for change. Both presbyopes ('old-age' sight) and true far-sighted hyperopes (where the eyeball is foreshortened) are wearing magnification lenses which make the world larger. These glasses can be reduced for close work to the same degree that short-sighted glasses are reduced. The usual standard for close vision is the Rosenbaum card, a close version of the distance chart. On it is a line of print corresponding to 20/40 in the distance. Obtain a pair of reading glasses which give you clarity on that line *only*, not on anything larger. Or you might want to obtain glasses with which the letter size you generally use is readable but blurry. Your eye practioner can help you with this.

If you have an antique collection of your old reading glasses around the house you might be able to go back to the weaker ones using your own judgment. This is only advisable if they are single lens (not bifocals) and contain no astigmatic correction, or color tint.

Consider doing without reading glasses altogether. Release the old habits of reading for a time to give your eyes some space for improvement. Take a walk instead of reading, visit a friend, go to the art gallery or museum. Guide yourself through this book slowly and softly. Activate the ideas in the following chapters. Then absorb the meaning of the Thrill of the Great White glow in chapter 14 to clear up your reading blur.

THE ASTIGMATISM GOES

From a natural vision point of view it is best if all the astigmatic correction is removed from your glasses right away. Sometimes this is not possible when it accompanies other types of refractive error or is high. In this case, cooperative eye practitioners have in the past reduced the astigmatism by half or as much as possible (they juggle it with myopic correction for example) to achieve 20/40 under-corrected vision.

Many eye practitioners will generally not even give a correction for low degrees of astigmatism (½ to one diopter) whereas others will put in correction at the smallest sign of it. Practitioners who prescribe soft contact lenses know that they cannot correct the lower degrees of astigmatism so they generally ignore its presence altogether. This practice rarely produces any negative symptoms.

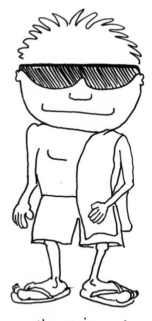

BIFOCALS, CONTACTS, SUNGLASSES

Bifocals are one pair of glasses with two different corrections. Even with the new cosmetically invisible line, the fact that you have one correction on the top and another on the bottom means that part of the time you are looking through the wrong lens. These invisible bifocals also produce distortions in side vision. This sets up strain in your seeing. It is better to use two pairs of glasses than one bifocal pair. If you are myopic enough to be dependent on glasses you will probably end up in bifocals as your ability to accommodate diminishes. In this case again it is better to have two pairs of transition glasses, one for distance, one for close, or leave off reading for a time as suggested above.

Contacts are *seductive* in several ways. Firstly there are no heavy obscuring frames on the face. Secondly, some high myopes can be optically corrected more easily with contacts. The disadvantages are that they deprive the eyes of oxygen, they must be kept scrupulously clean, and they cannot be taken off and on as easily as glasses. And from an organic point of view they are still a foreign object in the eye. As you activate the natural vision improvement games in your life it is advisable to use glasses rather than contact lenses. As energy and life return to your eyes you may not tolerate the contacts as well.

Once you have raised your acceptance of light through 'Sunning' in Chapter 8, you'll no longer have a need for sunglasses. Also the tints in glasses can adversely affect your brain functioning. If you are in extreme glare situations the pinhole spectacles are a possibility.

... the tints in glasses can affect your brain functioning

PINHOLE SPECTACLES

Pinhole spectacles are not glasses at all, nor is the idea of reducing light anything new. Eskimos in 'white out' snow conditions used to carve goggles of wood with a narrow horizontal slit across the front. This allowed them to travel in an environment where light was coming from every direction and all contours were missing. If that Eskimo had been myopic (not many Eskimos were, until they started going to school), she/he might also have seen more clearly. The clarity given by the pinholes is due to the fact that the blur circle on the retina is reduced.

This figure depicts what occurs when pinhole spectacles are placed in front of a myopic eye looking at a distant object:

1. Parallel light entering this (short-sighted) eye is brought to a focus within the eye (F) and produces a large blur circle on the retina.

2. The moment a pinhole is introduced in front of the eye a much narrower parallel pencil of light comes through the hole. The light again goes through the focal point F resulting in a much smaller blur circle on the macular area.

People with both close and distant blur, and astigmatism, are able to use pinhole spectacles as T-glasses while they're in the process of improving their sight through natural means. Pinholes have some disadvantages. They are not useful at night nor recommended for driving. They reduce peripheral vision and most driving laws require compensatory lenses. One of their greatest advantages is that they are not prescriptive. Almost everyone, no matter what their error of refraction, sees clearly through the holes. In addition, they encourage saccadic motion. Staring through them is unusually counterproductive. Using the pinholes temporarily for reading, TV viewing, and theatre going is very handy. They are inexpensive in comparison to prescriptive glasses.

It is important if you do obtain pinholes to use as T-glasses that you give yourself some time to adjust to them. They have a honeycomb effect that is distracting at first if the eyes are extremely decentralized (see chapter 11). Put them on, do some yawning, edging from Chapter 6, and blinking until your brain says. 'This super clear vision is all right'. At this point the brain stops paying attention to the black occluding plastic and tunes into the messages coming through the pinholes.

An opthalmologist recommends using the pinhole effect—'when you lose your eyeglasses in the woods, try viewing through a pinhole. Vision will be improved. Pinhole glasses would be used more frequently except that they decrease the illumination and the field of vision: (Steven Goldberg, M.D.: *Ophthalmology Made Ridiculously Simple*, p.12.). Perhaps Dr Goldberg does not realize there may be a more intriguing reason why pinholes are not used more. They have in fact been harshly suppressed by legal means in several countries. Thanks to the persistance of an Australian woman living in California, who spent $70,000 in legal fees to keep her product

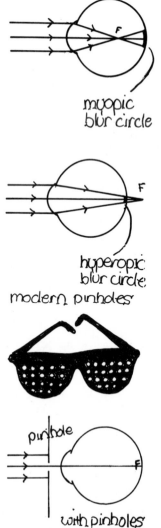

myopic
blur circle

hyperopic
blur circle

modern pinholes

pinhole

with pinholes

Stepping Out of Glasses

available through health food stores, the pinholes can be obtained. See 'OTHER RESOURCES', p.206.

APPROACHING THE PROFESSIONALS

Invariably when I mention reducing glasses, anxious faces appear. 'How will you get anybody to do it?' 'My eye doctor laughed in my face when I mentioned it.' Yet in every city in the world where I have taught there have been willing and interested (if not outright supportive) eye doctors and optometrists who will weaken glasses. Remember the following notions when you ask someone to reduce your prescription.

1. The eye practitioners are there to serve you.
2. They are not legally obliged to prescribe glasses stronger than 20/40 or 20/33, or 6/12.
3. Most eye practitioners (with some exceptions), are not trained in or exposed to the concepts of self-healing and alternative methods. Tell them what you require and bring to them your understanding of these concepts.
4. Ask your practitioner to support the possibility of rapid improvement by giving you the least possible correction. There is room for the doctor's option in this matter. Sometimes professional skepticism tends to cast a dark cloud over vision students' enthusiasm. Never mind. It is your vision and your project.
5. Do the relaxation activity described in chapter 4 before and after handling the technical aspect of weakened glasses and the necessary journey to the practitioner.
6. Wear your T-glasses (the prescriptive ones) if you have a restriction on your drivers' license. Wear T-glasses or pinholes if your livelihood requires a certain minimal visual acuity, such as typing, reading dials, labels, coaching, etc. Make sure your prescriptive T-glasses have no tint, color, prisms, or special treatment. It is especially recommended that the frames be plastic rather than metal so that energy flows (meridians) through the head area are not short-circuited by the metal.

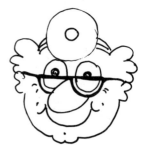

There are willing and interested optometrists

People sometimes complain at the prospect of buying how many? pairs of reduced lenses. Yet they often spend scads on updated stronger ones. It is possible to use your current frames and simply have the lenses changed.

It is important that you reduce your glasses and do not wear strong correction (they can be over-correcting you after five minutes of relaxing activity), and that you do your natural vision improvement games even when you are wearing your T-glasses.

Let's say you have been wearing stepped down glasses with myopic correction in them. You use these glasses only for driving and very occasionally at a play or sports event. You've been activating some of the vision games into your life. You notice that when you do put the glasses on you get:

1. Headaches
2. A sensation that your eyeballs are being pulled forward.
3. Super sharp vision.

If any of these signs appear, get yourself another pair of reduced lenses as soon as possible. Wearing glasses that are too strong, even for a few seconds, pulls your physical eye to the curvature of the glass lenses and causes terrific strain. Your pliable, adaptable living eyes will change and fluctuate, the glass will not.

Sometimes students go to pick up their reduced glasses and find that they are already seeing 20/20 through them. The eye doctor, softened by astonishment, then sits down and gives the person a further reduction on the spot. Nothing can keep an avid vision student from progressing like putting on a pair of glasses that are too strong.

Your clarity of vision lasts as long as you maintain and enjoy your new relaxed habits. If you find that you are able to function efficiently and happily in your life, pass your drivers' test, read easily, there is no longer a need to wear eyeglasses for any purpose. The excellent visual habits you will have acquired to escape from glasses are yours for the rest of your life.

Of course if you revert back to your old, tense, unbalanced ways, then eyeglasses will probably reappear on your nose. Even then, reviving your knowledge and experience can bring you back your clarity, especially if you've been taking good care of yourself.

BRINGING VISION BACK TO LIFE

In the next three chapters we will explore and play with the main concepts of the Bates Theory: movement, imagery and light, adding some up-to-date ideas and confirmation of his brilliant insights. We are ready to move.

Chapter 6

Improving Vision with Movement

The eye movements that cause seeing to take place are constant small vibrations. Because these vibrations resemble the flicking of a (French) sail in the wind, they are called 'saccades'. The saccades do two things. Firstly they stimulate your retinal nerve cells with a continuous strobing light show. The optic nerves then flash the details of this show to the visual brain at the back of your head.

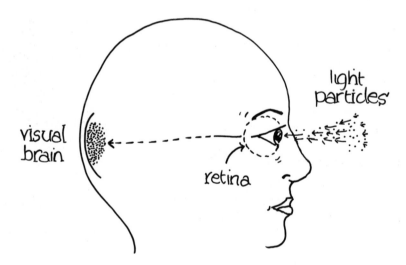

Secondly, the saccades sweep the light particles from your current *mental point of interest* into the keenest seeing part of your retina — the 'fovea centralis'. This action keeps your mind and eyes together and gives you sharp visual acuity.

When your eyes and attention pause on something, it may look like your eyes are stationary. But they are not. The saccadic dance continues, exciting your eyes, brain, and mind with the light energy that's bouncing about in your environment.

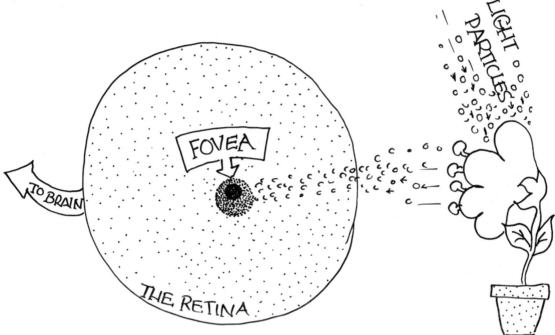

The saccades are speedy. Their duration is from two one-hundredths of a second to ten one-hundredths of a second. And they are short. They travel from two minutes of a degree to twenty minutes of a degree (a minute is 1/21,600 of a circle). The saccades are measured in parts of a circle because they actually occur as tiny rotations of the whole eyeball.

In the recording of an eye regarding the bust of Nefertiti we see how the saccadic motion causes a tracing of contours and an absorption of interesting details. The place where the lines change direction are the 'fixation' points — a misnomer because there the eyes vibrate the most, responding to small details of light and shadow.

If your saccadic movements were to completely stop, you would see nothing at all within three seconds. If the saccades were somehow slowed down, the energy flow through your eyes would drop and visual blur develop. When your saccadic dance is happening with no interferences of any kind, you are able to see clearly everywhere.

For you to further understand the connection between eye movements and the lowering of vision, I suggest you make some observations for yourself.

Notice the eyes of people with clear vision. Get up close to them and take a good look. You'll see their eyes actively hopping about in saccadic motion. The alert sparkling appearance of clear-seeing eyes comes from this freely flickering movement. Energetic active vision is happening in these eyes.

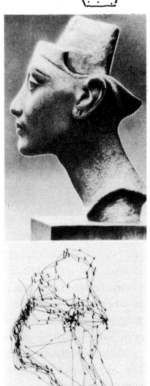

Improving Vision with Movement

Next find someone who wears strong glasses all the time. Ask them to remove their specs. You will notice the relative stillness of their eyes. Eyes with blurred vision take larger and fewer jumps. They appear to be less responsive, more subdued than clear-vision eyes.

A RECIPE FOR BLUR

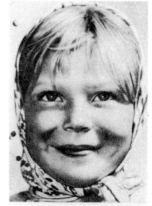

If you want to produce blur in a pair of otherwise healthy, clear-seeing eyes, slow down the saccadic dancing and cut down on energy flow in the body and mind. We humans have a simple method for impeding movement and high vibrations anywhere within us. We unconsciously tighten a few muscles and breathe in a restricted fashion. This holding response can become a habit. When it creeps into the visual system, it is called staring.

Habitual staring results in tight eye muscles, slowed saccadic activity, reduced energy flow through your eyes. It will put glasses on your nose sooner or later.

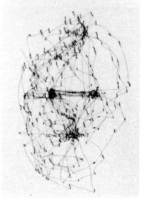

If your vision is blurred with refractive error right now, somewhere, at some time, you adopted a stare. Perhaps you noticed and perhaps not.

Maintaining a stare ties up a lot of energy. To perpetuate one unconscious stare for long periods of time you have to control your breath, making sure you do not breathe too deeply. You must hold your neck and shoulder muscles rigid and take care you don't laugh too often. You must park your eyes in one spot so that your eye movements are restricted. During all this your mind can either space out, try very hard to solve the unsolvable or just plain worry.

Staring and its resulting blur can be adopted as an excellent coping device at any time in life. You could have taken it on to deal with childhood stresses, illness, accidents. You might have used it to adapt to school, high-pressure job or a difficult emotional situation.

ARMS TOO SHORT?

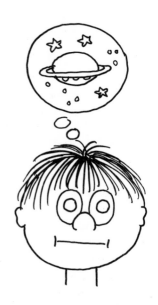

The aging process in the body, plus ignorance of how to reverse that process and our cultural programming has most people over age forty-five reaching for a pair of magnifiers. Therefore instead of relaxing and activating the eyes when reading blur comes on, most people start up a good stare. Trying to see the morning paper or phone book results in a quick trip to the 'old age' glasses. In chapter 14, Clear Easy Reading, you will learn ways to reverse and avoid the reading glasses trap.

Myopic (short-sighted) people are accomplished distance starers. The hyperopic and presbyopic (long-sighted) folks stare and strain beautifully up close. Astigmatics (those with corneas or lenses with aberrant curvature) do it at various angles.

Whatever the initial reason, distance, or time of onset, once into staring, you had to grope around for or were beneficently given (for a price) a fine pair of compensatory eyeglasses. The artificial lenses of eyeglasses are designed to help you manoeuvre adequately about the world. They also leave your initial blur and stare intact. Sometimes they make matters worse.

There is another way to go. You are able to reverse the habit of unconscious staring and allow your saccadic movements to re-establish their speed and number. This is accomplished through learning and using the Vision Movement Games.

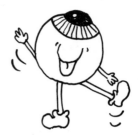

vision games

THE VISION MOVEMENT GAMES

At the beginning of this century, Dr Bates, with a twinkle in his eye, suggested that people start 'swinging' — moving their minds and bodies in a rhythmical fashion to free their eyes from staring and blur.

I prefer to call these various swings and all the vision improvement activities in this book, *games* rather than eye exercises. The word 'exercise' connotes work and goals. Blurred eyes are already overburdened with tension and dutiful exertion. To transform blur to clarity, we want your eyes to experience relaxation and pleasure. Gentle pleasant stimulation of your visual system will be far more effective than hours of determined effortful eye exercises.

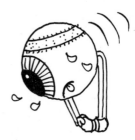

NOT exercises !

THE MAGIC PENCIL

Your pretend magic nose pencil extends and pulls in automatically

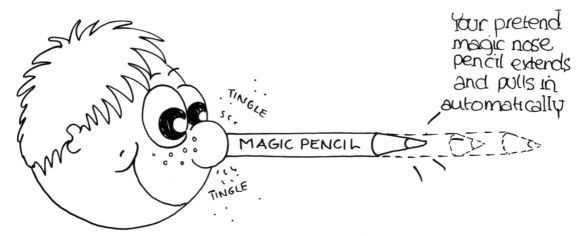

Sit in a quiet comfortable place. Give yourself credit for having been a successful starer. Notice what your stare is like. Emphasize it. Note your body state and current breathing style.

Realize and acknowledge that any energy you've tied up in staring you are now able to release into looseness, pleasure and play. Looseness is fostered by breathing fully.

Completely *exhale* every bit of air from your lungs by blowing out through your mouth. *Inhale* through your nose. Allow your tummy and your chest to expand. *Exhale* again through your mouth. Allow this new fullness of breathing to continue. Spontaneous yawns may arise. Please allow them expression.

Massage the tip end of your nose until it is warm, rosy and tingly.

Pretend you have a magic pencil that automatically extends and pulls in. This pencil is lighter than air.

Fasten the magic pencil to the tingling tip of your nose. The visual artist, you, has arrived.

Draw loosely the outlines of objects around you with the tip end of your magic pencil. Your mind relies on the shapes, borders, lines and edges — areas of high contrast, to define what it sees. Move your whole head as you sketch. Spend a few moments outlining large objects that you see best. Proceed to smaller shapes. Cycle from large to small shapes for a time, letting yourself become accustomed to this new activity and mobility.

Next, loosely draw shapes that are near and far. Your mental and visual attention is with the *end* of your magic pencil. The end of your pencil is soft. Your shoulders and neck release. Your whole body relaxes. You yawn widely and then you yawn some more.

Start *connecting* the objects in your environment with the pencil. Your sketching action and attention flow from one thing to another. Trace your hand, then a plant, a window, other objects *loosely, slowly.*

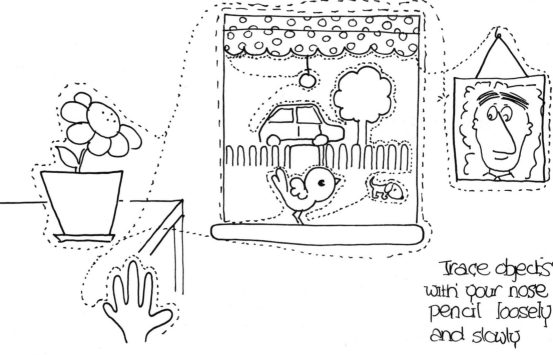

Trace objects with your nose pencil loosely and slowly

Your conscious mind is too slow to keep up with or order the saccadic movements around. These movements are automatic, subconscious, belonging more to the family of abilities that are generated from the 'imaging' right-brain. Adopting the nose pencil will keep your conscious mind in its own area of ability which is to notice, name, compare and appreciate.

As you intentionally relax with rhythmic drawing and edging, the rapid saccades will re-enter the scene by themselves.

... as you relax the saccades will re-enter the scene by themselves

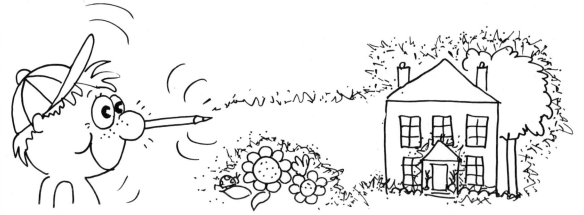

Your pencil adjusts automatically to distance or close. Being finicky or precise is passé here. You feel serene, regal, content. Relaxing blinks will appear to accompany your fluid movements.

Notice how much the world is on the go. Shapes and colors slide about as you sketch. Your eyes and mind are rejoicing in this new freedom of motion. Saccadic dancing is returning. You're playing with the visual.

Acknowledge yourself as a visual artist. Artists use light, color and shape to create images. You use these same elements to create eyesight within yourself.

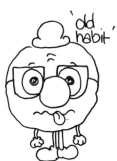

Staring is an unconscious habit. We transform habits by replacing them with more enjoyable beneficial habits.

Adopt the magic pencil as your lifelong friend. Your new habit is *sketching* with your pencil everywhere you go. *In private:* draw big and breathe big to release your eyes, neck and shoulders. *Stretch your arms* and yawn. Draw the shapes of your interiors, your visitors, TV characters, your horticulture, your personal culture.

In public: be subtle in your sketching, discreet in breathing deep. Enjoy colors and details of every environment you are in. Your continuous movement, *no matter how small*, will help you stay in communication with your surroundings.

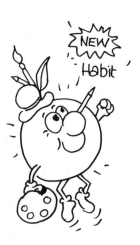

Facing other people: be a portraitist. With your nose pencil sketch mildly the other person's countenance. Move gently from eye to eye, to the mouth, around the halo of their hair. Blink and feel calm. You are deliberately imitating the way eyes saccadically take in faces. (See reproduction from *Eye Movements and Vision* by Alfred Yarbus on pp. 47 and 48.) This 'conversation swing' allows you to relate easily to other people's energy. You are not pinning them to the wall with your 'eye contact' — you are enjoying the touch of another's eyes.

On the road: driving is an important time to be visually alert and mentally grounded. If you have a glasses restriction on your drivers' licence you can legally wear a 20/40 correction. Wearing lenses reduced to this level will keep you safe on the road and still give your eyes room to change. Even when wearing your 20/40s it is important that you keep up your easy relaxing movements. Utilize the time in the car for establishing your new habits.

With your nose pencil *sketch and outline* the cars in front of you. *Trace* road signs. *Scan* from right to left. This *side to side* motion will be short to fit the roadway as it narrows off into the distance.

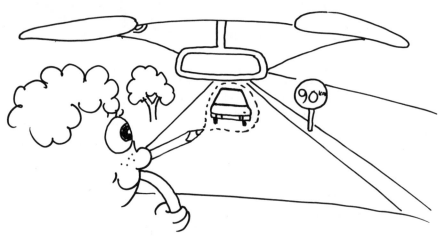

With your nose pencil sketch and outline the cars infront of you

This continuous relaxed scanning movement while traveling will allow you to register any vehicles or creatures that might move suddenly into your visual field. In fact, any motion across the outer edges of your retina stimulates a reflex to your brain that says, 'Hey, let's turn our head and get some direct information on this thing that just crept up on us.' This quick visual responsiveness can be inhibited by spaced-out staring. Your 'motoring swing' will keep you alert and improve your vision at the same time.

NEAR-FAR IN THE CAR

If you are making a long freeway trip where there are vistas stretching out in front of you and little traffic, it is valuable and fun to do a *near-far* movement to further turn on your vision.

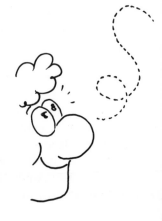

With your magic pencil slide your attention down/out the center line of the highway to the vanishing point. There you sketch the distant shapes for a moment. Then *slide* your attention back in on the centre line to the front of your car. Circle briefly and slide into the distance once more. Repeat this sequence, inhaling and exhaling with the rhythm of your movement. Be loose with this activity. Adapt it as you please. Your head will tilt up slightly as your attention goes outward. It will come down slightly as your attention comes inward. This action maintains a flexible neck. Your eyes are blinking easily. Your brain is getting plenty of oxygen from your full breathing. You stay awake and attentive. Your vision has an excellent chance to clear. If you are wearing T-glasses lenses, this movement may give you superkeen vision through those glasses. If you are not wearing glasses this *near-far* action may give you prolonged flashes of bright detailed vision.

This near-far swing is meant to be done at other times and places. The principle is the same, rocking your attention into the distance and up close again, whether you are sitting at the beach, in your garden or in the office. You may use an imaginary rope, a kite string, a long chain of pearls to help guide your attention in and out. It is excellent for both short and far-sightedness. The myopes roll their relaxed close vision outward. The hyperopes roll their easy clear far vision from the distance into their body's vicinity. Do it with eyes closed for a while, then with eyes open (not in the car unless you are a passenger!) We will meet up with the near-far swing again in Chapter 14, the chapter on reading.

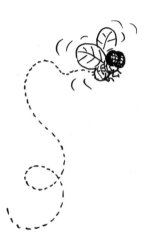

WHAT IF IT MOVES?

We have discussed the vision movement games in relation to objects that are sitting 'still'. What about things that move? Things like Pac-persons gobbling dots, tennis, foot and squash balls, circling hawks and nice people. Simply follow these moving objects with your nose. Move your whole head. You need not outline a moving object because its motion will automatically attract and carry your attention along with it.

SOOTHING SIMPLE PENCIL PLAY

Create a calm place in your environment. Sit or lie down in that spot and *close your eyes.*

Reaffirm the presence of your magic pencil on the end of your nose. Allow your thoughts to drain away. Allow your breath to deepen.

Imagine and sketch the simplest shape possible, a circle, for instance. Draw it several times. Let associations related to circles percolate up from your memory banks. Sketch the images that develop.

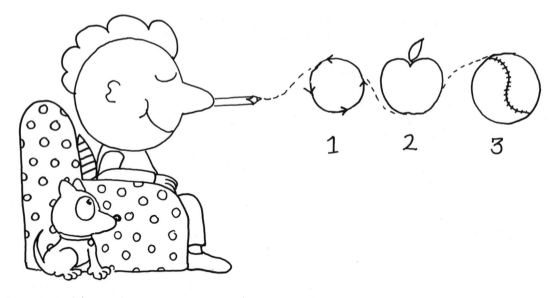

1 2 3

Let your circle change into an apple (a beach ball, a bicycle wheel).
Then draw a rectangle and let it turn into a house (jack-in-the-box,
Rubik's cube). | Continue drawing other simple shapes and turn them
into familiar objects.

Notice that your eyes are being encouraged to relax and vibrate.
Your breathing has become more regular and full. You may feel
backed-up yawns arising. Open your mouth and let those yawns
have their day.

Open your eyes and continue sketching for a while. Drink in
the refreshed colors and newly unveiled details of your visual world.
Stretch and yawn some more.

UPRIGHT CLARITY WITH THE FEATHER

Stand calmly and confidently in the center of a room or outdoors
in a spacious area. Your feet are shoulder width apart, your arms
relaxed at your sides.

Listen to some rhythmical music or call up some deep inner humming of your own.

Shift your weight lazily from one foot to the other. Your whole
body sways gently from side to side; go slowly at first to get
accustomed to this new feeling of space. Later, move with more
vigor and élan.

Place a long, gorgeous, magic, imaginary feather on the end
of your nose. (Put your nose pencil in your pocket for now.)

Dust the world with your magic feather moving from side to
side. Visual shapes and colors will slide by, giving you an increasing

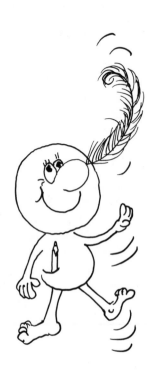

sense of motion. Sometimes it may appear that the world is gliding by in the opposite direction. This contributes to the general happy dancing that's happening in your eyes, mind, and your physical world.

Tickle the floor or grass with your feather. Tickle the walls or bushes with your feather. Keep moving and flowing with your feather. Gradually you will feel changes happening within you. Any one of the following cues will indicate that you have shifted toward deep relaxation within your visual system:

1. Spontaneous yawning with watering eyes.
2. Your mind softens and broadens.
3. Your face feels softer and broader.
4. Colors and details brighten and clear.
5. Your depth perception intensifies.
6. You become visual as well as verbal, seeing catches up with thinking.
7. You feel simple, content, connected, centered, serenely alive.

Continue the feather swing as long as you like. Carry the resulting relaxation with you through the entire day.

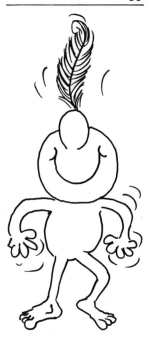

FREE AS A BIRD

This is another option for a standing vision game. With a daring leap of fancy, imagine you are a bird — an eagle, hawk or owl, or perhaps you would like to be an ocean-going gull or osprey. Visualize your 'birdness'. First with eyes closed, later with eyes open.

You are standing and swaying. Imagine the planet earth from the viewpoint of the bird that you are. Become freer with your body, freer with your movements as you bring the spirit and perceptions of the bird into your self.

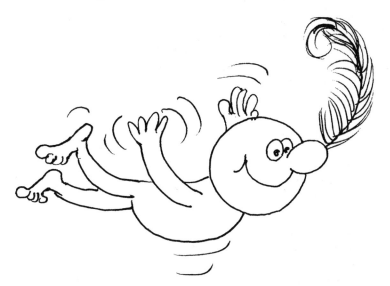

...Bring the spirit and perceptions of the bird into your self

Bend your whole body. Flex your limbs, soar with your arms. Let your head and nose feather move at random. You are naturally graceful as you sweep across the imagined domains of the aerial creatures. *Fly* over vast deserts, mountain ranges, oceans. *Improvise* this game to the edges of your imagination. *Move* any part of your body that is asking to express itself. Your eyes will love it all and respond with plenty of saccadic twinkles. *Yawn, Yawn, Yawn.* Eventually come in for a landing. Open your eyes gently and allow the physical objects around you to reconnect with your mind and attention. Let the relaxation you have gained from your 'bird' experience flow with you into the next activity of the day.

THE LANGUAGE OF CLEAR VISION

The words you use in both talking and thinking have the ability to turn vision off and to turn vision on. Phrases such as '*try* to see', 'I *can't* see it', and 'I *lost* my vision' tend to perpetuate a lack of subconscious visual energy. Because your mind and physical eyes are intimately connected, vision is an extremely suggestible function. Fortunately it works both ways. What you are able to turn off, you are able to turn on. Therefore your language is a powerful ally in your vision improvement project. Let's find and put together some words and phrases that will influence your subconscious mind and your physical vision.

Here is a list of words natural vision students have associated with their staring habit and a list describing the transformation of the stare.

With your magic nose feather lightly scan up and down the left column of words. Do any of these descriptions look familiar? If so, suspend all judgement about them and about yourself. The states of being described by these words are neither good nor bad, right nor wrong. They are demonstration states which reveal to us the possibilities of their opposites. We wouldn't be able to appreciate the value of the second column unless we have become familiar with the first.

**The Staring
Blurred Eyes Are:**
absent
foggy
fixed
spaced out
dim
dull
rigid
tense

**The Mobile
Clear Eyes Are:**
present
clear
loose
grounded
bright
keen
agile
relaxed

hard	soft
distracted	'with it'
blank	full
empty	brimming
stiff	flexible
unconscious	aware
holding	released
scared	secure
dead	alive
flat	sparkling
despairing	happy
hostile	friendly
cold	warm
indifferent	loving
distant	giving
severe	smiling
contracted	expansive
opaque	transparent
aggressive	receptive
scattered	connected
static	energetic
nervous	confident
constrained	free
trying to see	seeing

Add your own words to the list, reflecting your experience and observations.

Now let's play with the words in the right column. Slide your white nose feather (they come in all colors) up and down these vision-fostering words. Let your mind and body absorb the energy, attitude and pleasure of these word states. Imagine that these words are knocking on the door of your visual creative brain. They're inviting all your best energies out to play in the physical universe. With all these alive, positive optimistic parts of yourself consistently activated, you will be able to transform yourself into a clear 'see-er'.

One effective way to utilize the language of clear vision is to make up new lines for yourself in the theater of your everyday life. Replace the old negative thoughts such as 'eyesight can't be changed' and 'I'm too old' or 'my vision is too far gone' with a new script that you make up right here on the spot.

Find the words in the right column that mean the most to you now. Put your word choices into the spaces below and say the resulting sentence to yourself a few times. Do this until this new thought has 'jelled' inside you. Let these thoughts prevail through the day. Speak them aloud to others. Whisper them to yourself.

'My eyes are_____right now.'
'My vision is_____today.'
'My attitude is_____all the time.'
'My mind is_____consistently'.
'My_____is_____everywhere.'

These phrases are suggestions. Find something that feels right to you and use it to counteract your negative thought patterns. Convince the negatives that they are no longer welcome in your mind by overriding them with one of your new positives. Movement, flexibility, a visual language and clear seeing become a natural part of you.

You have now acquired some experience with improving your vision through movement and language. Taking your new 'art of seeing' materials with you, let's move on to the lore of improving vision with imagery.

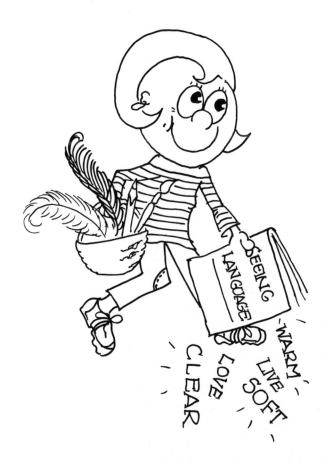

Chapter 7

Improving Vision with Imagery

It is our imagination that weaves the messages flowing into the visual brain into rich dimensional fabric of our seeing. Without active continuous image-making in the mind, the nerve input to the visual cortex remains rudimentary and lifeless.

When the ability to imagine is pushed low on the cultural priority list, both creativity and eyesight deteriorate. Such comments as 'Oh, that's just your imagination' probably curbed some wonderful creative and visual adventures.

The emphasis on identifying eyesight with black and white verbal performance has presented another challenge to free and easy vision. People become locked into thinking of their eyesight in terms of letters and numbers. If at any time you were unable to read the black on white letters on the flat eyechart you had 'bad' vision forever. Your wonderful imaging power may have rusted in the closet for lack of respect and recognition. Many beginning students over the years have averred to me that they 'have no imagination'. Yet everyone does or we would not be seeing at all.

Now it may be time for you to open that closet door!

When you visualize and imagine, your right 'seeing' hemisphere of the brain turns on. If it is switched on and sharing perceptual tasks with the verbal analytical left brain, then all functions of mind and body become easier. This combination of spontaneous imaging and sensible thinking will give us maximum well-being in all areas of our life. We will delve into this more deeply in chapter 12.

Ingredients from your memory banks, your dreams, your creativity, all the known and unknown, conscious and unconscious landscapes are accessible territory for your imagination.

To attend to, develop and connect imagery to vision will increase your ability to see more clearly. Image making in the mind actually governs the shaping of saccadic movement patterns. Alfred Yarbus said at the conclusion of his book that a person's eyes will generally move around whatever the mind is interested in. The way

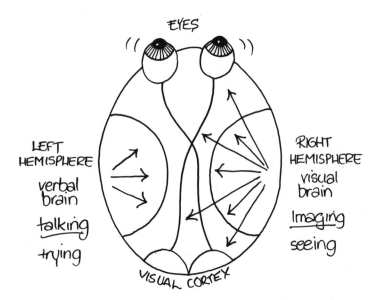

a person 'thinks' determines which details of a scene the eyes will dance around.

If you are a carpenter and go into the woods, you'll see the trees in relation to the lumber you could cut, your eyes seeking out the girth and height of the trees. A biologist will notice and see the birds, the wildlife, the shape of the leaves, and a conservationist may see the relationship of the trees to each other, to the stream nearby, to the cloud formations overhead. The eyes will physically move together and 'see' a certain version of the same 'real' forest in accordance with these varied mental interests.

If you close your eyes and imagine a tree, the eyes will move in their saccadic jumps just as if you had your eyes open examining an oak in front of you.

For this reason, it is wonderful to turn on your imaging powers in the restful state of closed eyes. This will result in relaxation of body and mind which you will be able to transfer to opened eyes in more and more settings (including the office where the eyechart sits). Eventually we want to be imagining all the time whether eyes are open or closed. When we do this there is a continuous flow of energy through your right hemisphere into the left brain, an integration process that replaces the tedious work of trying to see with the effortless seeing of relaxed natural vision.

Give yourself a demonstration of these two 'styles' of seeing first without imagining and then *with*.

'I am now sketching the outline of a book over there in the bookshelf. The book is *out there*; it is not inside me in any way. In fact I borrowed that book. It doesn't belong to me. Am I just imagining that book? No way. Do you think I'm crazy? I see it.

It's over there and very blurry, even though I'm sketching away like mad here with this "nose pencil".'

'I am now sketching the outline of the book that I'm imagining in my bookshelf. I am painting the book green in my mind. The book actually exists in the back of my head. It's now brightening up and getting clearer. It's coming alive. Maybe it will sit up and start to talk to me. Perhaps it will tell me a story. I feel calm and content as I imagine and *see* this book.'

Choose other objects in your room. Do your magic pencil sketching while you do the above demonstrations a few times. Contrast trying to see something 'out there' with seeing while imagining in your mind. Once you have an awareness of this relaxed style of seeing you will be able to integrate it into your daily activities, occasionally murmuring 'I am imagining this' while you sketch your visual world'.

THE GROWTH AND DEVELOPMENT OF IMAGINATION

People with blurred vision have given me three kinds of responses to the suggestion that they promote their imagery to clear their vision. A small group of people will say with a tinge of defensiveness, 'I'm an artist and I have great visual imagination.' If you are one of these visualizing, artistic people, it is important that you realize your ability to imagine is not being questioned. What is needed is that it gets 'hooked' up to your physical seeing process.

The second larger group love to sit back and be told colorful stories. They like to tape record their vision lessons and are content to have their mental pictures stimulated by the teacher's voice. This group misses the realization that they too have the ability to stimulate their own internal images. Tape recordings are recommended to start with. Then one day dip a mental toe into your own pool of memories to create a self-spun story.

The third group of students respond with rocky resistance to the whole message. They either assert that imagination is not necessary to vision or that they themselves have no imagination. The folk in this group who eventually soften up and turn on their power of imagery experience profound personal changes in their perception and personality.

The following imagery games are designed with all three of the above groups in mind, and for anyone else who desires to awaken and develop their inner and outer seeing.

The imagination retreats in the face of judgment and putdown. It responds beautifully to invitation and modest amounts of encouragement.

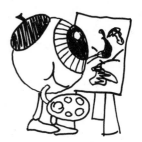

Improving Vision with Imagery

When you visualize, draw the images with your nose pencil or paintbrush so that you maintain a small movement all the time. When you finish with a specific imagery activity and are ready to resume your ordinary activities, *ground* yourself.

GROUNDING

Clasp both hands together and squeeze them tightly as you exhale completely through your mouth. Your feet are magnets and the earth is metal. Open your eyes gently and blink a few times. The grounding action will keep your mind in your body and help to integrate your visual calmness into any environment.

Preparing the Field

Sit or *lie down* comfortably and close your eyes. The darkness that you see is your visual territory. You are the caretaker, gardener and harvester of this inner space. You have free rein to plant, grow, produce and arrange colors, shapes and details. Let's explore this dark region for a while until you feel totally at home in your own field.

Ask your thinking mind to quieten. Let your thoughts thin out. In a quiet space between two thoughts move into the darkness before your eyes.

Do you see greys and dark shapes rolling about? This is a great field of fertile loam. Anything will grow here. Enjoy the nothingness, the undefinable that preludes specific form. Let the bare toes of your mind delight in the dark rich potential of your visual field. Notice how low your field extends. And how high. Explore the sides to the right and to the left. Does your field have perimeters or does

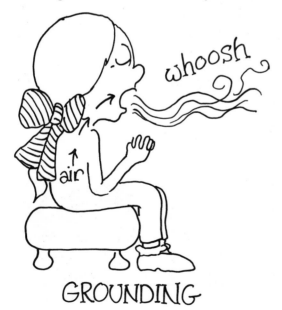

GROUNDING

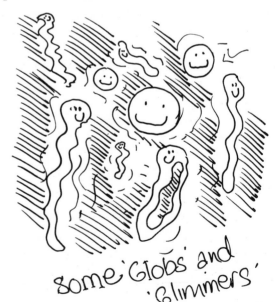

some 'Globs' and 'Glimmers'

it go on forever? Now plumb the depths of your field. How deep does this dark soil lie? You're taking an independent journey through the warm darkness of your inner vision beyond your usual mental pathways.

Now let us turn to globs and glimmers. Have you seen a *Glob?* Globs are fairly common in these parts. They float here and there through the darkness. They are indefinite, meaningless, quiet. You'll see them at times when you are peaceful inside, allowing yourself to experience the unknown and unnameable.

Now some *Glimmers* come around. The glimmers could be retinal afterimages that occur when you open and close your eyes. Appreciate their will-o-the-wisp quality as they waft across your field. Play a simple game with the glimmers. If you sweep your nose feather from side to side, the glimmers will slide in the opposite direction from your movement. This action will bring on a lovely releasing shadow play in your dark visual field.

Let's begin now to name some of the globs and glimmers. This defining left brain action will ease you into connecting your verbal and visual brains without having the first elbow out the second. Whimsy will help keep things in balance.

One of your glimmers has turned into a spiral? That's good. Trace the spiral with your nose as far as it goes. My current glob has turned into a black box. Wonder what's in it? With my nose I shall carefully lift the lid — out pops an iridescent yellow butterfly. *Play* with your shapes for a while, edging and naming them.

One of my afterimages has become a red laser beam. (Have you noticed how you can make vague shapes instantly become something definite just by naming them?) We might use my scarlet laser beam to paint a glorious sunset in the desert. Now, what's happening in your field?

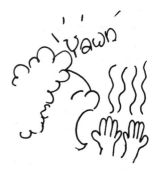

FERTILIZING BY HAND — PALMING

Let's enrich our visual fields by *palming.* Hold your hands, palms up, in front of you. Breathe deeply feeling the air expanding your tummy. Yawn several times. Do this until you sense energy vapors rising from the palms of your hands. Your hands are powerful transmitters of healing, warmth and spirit Place the center of your slightly cupped palms over the centre of your eyes, closing off all outside light. There is a little space between your palms and your eyeballs. Your fingers may overlap on your forehead. Lie down, your elbows extending straight to the sky. Or, sit with your arms supported. A more profound darkness may appear if you close your eyes. The energy and warmth flowing through your hands will soften tight eye and facial muscles. Your brain circuits will drink in the beneficial power streaming through your hands.

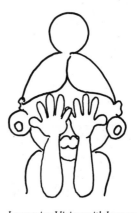

Improving Vision with Imagery

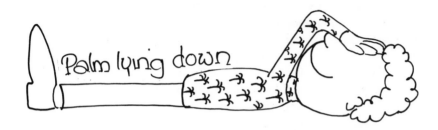

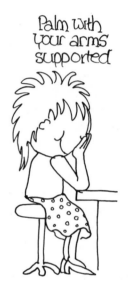

Palm with your arms supported

While palming, *imagine* a blue sun in the center of the earth. Cobalt, ultramarine, and indigo hues are emanating from this sun. The blue colors radiate up through the layers of the earth to your feet. This brilliant strong light flows up through your feet into your legs. It is a colored river of energy that carries health, vitality and balance into your body and mind. The river moves up through your torso into your chest. Your lungs respond by filling totally with fresh oxygen and by exhaling every iota of old air. The blue flows into your shoulders. Here it is absorbed by your shoulder muscles which expand from the inside. The blue river divides and flows into your arms. Feel the vibrant calming energy in your muscles, veins and bones. The blue light streams into your hands. Here it pauses for a time, building up its energy, swirling in the centre of your palms. Instinctively you will know the right moment to release the blue energy into your eyes. A flood of magical light and joy pours into your eyes and brain. Let it soak into the bones of your face, into the tissues and cells of your eyes. It brings healing, vitality and clarity to your whole visual system.

Imagine the blue light flowing to the visual centres in the back of your head. The seeing cells of your visual brain awaken and buzz with color and aliveness. Finally visualize the blue light expanding through and around the back of your head. Keeping your eyes closed, bring your palms away from your eyes slowly. Give a big stretch and a yawn. Put your magic feather on the end of your nose and begin tickling the room around you. When you feel ready, *open* your eyes and enjoy the freshness and vitality of your vision.

When palming there is no outside light stimulating your visual system. Therefore the light that your imagination employs to create the colored images in your visual field comes from your own internal lighting department. If you haven't called upon your lighting crew for some time, be patient. They will soon be producing some wonderful visual effects for you.

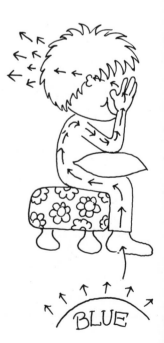

BLUE

THE RECEPTIVE STATE

You will also notice that we often *ask* for images to appear in the vision improvement games. Images arise spontaneously from the unknown (right hemisphere) with no trying, forcing or pushing by the conscious mind. It follows that *asking for* an image is one of the most effective ways to increase imaginative production. In my experience, insistently pushing or trying to force images or memories to appear puts you right into blankness and frustration. After *asking for*, the next step is to be *receptive*.

1. Make a direct request of your imagination, your subconscious mind, 'Dear Imagination, please send me the image of a peacock with its tailfeathers spread.'
2. Now drop all directives, expectations and verbal afterthoughts.
3. Be happy with *whatever* images your imagination sends you even if the first pictures look more like ravens.

IMAGE PLUS MOTION

Palm with your eyes closed. Put the magic pencil on the end of your nose and sketch an apple tree in the centre of your visual field. *Draw* the greyish trunk with its branches stretching up in the clear blue sky. *Draw* the fingery roots extending down into the rich loamy earth. Add some apple green leaves. Ask your internal lighting crew for some terrific sunlight to flood the scene and illuminate the shiny red apples that gleam in the branches.

Imagine that you walk forward in your field right up to the tree. Smell the aroma of sun-warmed grass and leaves. Reach up and pluck a single crimson apple. Polish it on your sleeve and hold it up to the light. See your face reflected in its glowing surface. Sniff the apple and take a bite. Savor the crunch and the sweet juice that fills your mouth. Toss the apple up into the clear blue sky. Aha! It descends as a red rubber ball.

Throw the ball far into the distance. Follow it with your nose. It grows smaller and smaller until it disappears at the horizon. Call the ball back. It reappears — wherever — bouncing gaily towards you. Call it into your hands. Circle and examine it with your nose. Has it collected any marks of its journey? Is it ready to fly again? Does it want to leap and sparkle and cover great distance in a single bound? Let it. The red ball is your friend and is available any time, anywhere, to help you develop flexibility in your imagination and saccadic movement in your eyes.

Imagine you're in the Australian outback. Look at the boomerang in your hand. It is the color of red earth, white-painted with Aboriginal hieroglyphics and is about 60 centimetres long. Notice its aerodynamic shape, rather like the swept-back wings of a jet plane.

You are holding the boomerang by one end and its smooth warm wood feels snug in your grip. You raise it backwards over your shoulder. You throw. Watch it leap from your hand. Instantly the boomerang becomes a spinning blade scything through the air in a low flat trajectory. It speeds its way over the heads of the low

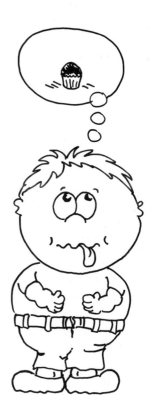

'Dear Imagination, please send me the image of a giant chocolate cake'

desert shrubs, shrinking ... getting smaller until it almost disappears into the sun-baked ruddy hills beyond.

Follow it as it rises now, soaring and banking like a bird. It arches back towards you; its motion a shimmer in the clear blue sky. Watch it growing larger ... coming closer ... you hold up your hand and see the boomerang slap into your palm. Its heartbeat stops and it lies there quiet and still.

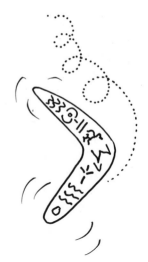

HARVESTING THE CROP

Now that you have experienced the dark fertile emptiness, the blue river of energy, color and movement in your visual imagination, it is time to see what visual treasures are lying around in your memory banks. Just below the surface of your conscious mind are the accumulations of your life's experience. Let us enjoy and utilize them for well-being and vision in the present.

I'm going to share with you some examples of memory bank stories that can be used while palming and imaging.

Following each experience related below I would like you to think of a story of your own and write it down.

Your own story is important to anchor your experience and to move through self-consciousness. Do it in your own fashion. Add a sketch as well. This will affirm your ability to use your own resources to improve your vision.

I am three. I'm standing in the sunlight on the road that parts the houses in the tiny village that is my world. Men came one day and put some black stuff called tar on our road. I'm walking barefoot through the warm glowing air in my red shorts and white top. Some other kids are with me. My older brother, Larry, the capable one, and three others. Big ones, and little ones, like me. We are walking on the side of the tar road past the white houses toward the green cornfields. The tar is getting hot and soft under my feet. It is soft grey and wavy in places. Ah, here something wonderful has happened. The tar has grown bubbles as big as my hand. Little soft black houses that bugs could live in. Let's all sit down at the side of the road and play with these bubbles, these pillowy interesting bumps. With my fingernail I make a hole in the side and lift. OOOh, it's black in there. And shiny. Gooey, pushey, soft and stretchy. The sunlight is shining right inside the little house. The wet tar in there is shiny black. Sticky, too. Look, it spreads. It's sticking to my knee and my fingers. And you have some in your hair and on your nose.

I am riding on a small ferry boat from the tip of the Yucatan Peninsula to an offshore island in the Caribbean Ocean. I see my hands resting on the white railing of the boat. Friendly sunlight splashes over me and spreads across the smooth sparkling water. Diamond clusters twinkle on the turquoise surface. The sky overhead is a softer blue, empty and spacious. I ask the peacefulness and beauty of water and sky to enter my mind.

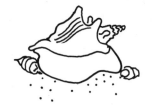

When the ferry halts at the wooden dock, I feel the granulated seashells massage the soles of my feet. I walk along the shore, welcoming the fresh ocean air into my body. A mound of shells sits by the side of a stream that slides into a lagoon. It takes two hands to lift one shell. It is as large as my head, chalky grey on the outside and smooth peachy-pink on the inside. With seeing fingertips I caress the shell, imagining what its home was like under the sea. The water heard me call its name and beckons. I wade into its coolness to the level of my hips. Iridescent pink and green fish flip their tails as I peek into their warm liquid domain. The lagoon is a transparent window into a tranquil expansive home of grainy white floors, furnished with red coral. A glowing purple fan coral undulates in the current — a living sculpture. 'Yes, you sprightly darting rainbow fishes, I will come and swim with you.' In the joy of this thought I pick up the shining water in my hands and fling it up into the sun, delighting in the cool sparkles sliding down my eyelids and cheeks.

I am standing on a street near the harbor. The sun is shining between grey scudding clouds. A brisk ocean breeze reddens my cheeks. A mammoth silver bus draws up to the curb. The descending figures must be Japanese tourists. Dark-suited gentlemen with black camera cases, pretty petite ladies in flowery dresses holding on to their hats, shiny black hair and brown eyes. These people mill around me as they gather images on retinas and Fushi paper. Soon they file neatly back into the bus. The bus motor starts up. I turn, glancing across the bus to an open window just above me. A woman looks towards me. Instantly a great wave of warmth flows between us. She gleams a quick 'hello' to me as a smile spreads across my face. We reach out our arms and brush fingertips as the bus glides away.

When I was at university, I went one evening to see an 'art' movie. In the huge cool lecture room I sat watching a three-hour long silent film called *Grass*. No sound, just a continuous collage of black and white images of a migrating tribe. Over vast plains of grasslands these patient people trudged. They traversed raging rivers where a precious goat was swept away in the frothy torrent. They scrambled through narrow mountain passes. Everyone helped each other. Men in turbans carried small children on their backs. Women in

long robes dispensed the meagre rations. I allowed myself to imagine having been on such a trek. Feeling my feet in their thin leather
sandals. Walking miles each day carrying minimal belongings on
my back. Waking each morning to vistas of sunlit, windswept
steppes that gave way to craggy mountains. I would breathe the
high thin air of chilling blue atmospheres. When I close my eyes
now I see the stoic brown weathered faces of the people. And then
my sight is flooded with the tall carpets of grass, undulating, billow-
ing, green grass that stretches away for miles.

I recall an episode in the *Wind in the Willows* that delighted me
when I read it long ago. Rat and Mole were lazing along in their
boat on the country river. No, they were actually looking for a
lost baby animal and had almost given up the search in despair.
Suddenly Mole sat up with an entranced look on his face. He was
hearing an extremely faint sound that wafted over the river. At first
Rat didn't know what to do. He figured Mole had completely spaced
out. Then he too was captivated by the wisps of magical sound
that issued from a green covered island in the middle of the river.
The musical strains evoked for the humble animals the beauty of
the place where all the animals come from and to whence they will
all return. Picking up the oars, the two creatures paddled toward
the source of the sound. They landed and proceeded cautiously into
the centre of the island. Their astounded eyes beheld a shimmering
form. They could see horns and hooves and felt themselves embrac-
ed by infinite goodness and love. After a timeless moment of
dreamspace the sound of the pipe ceased and the two rodent friends
snapped back into reality and found themselves being hugged by
the lost baby whom they carried joyously home.

I see before me the mantle clock that always rests on the old oak
side table. It sits on one of grandmother's starched lace doilys, il-
luminated by light pouring through the window. I trace its rounded
head and two flat side arms with my nose pencil. The glass cover
protects a white moonface with gold dots depicting the hours. The
ornate brass arms stretch out from the moon's nose to different lengths.
They haven't budged in years. They're pausing in time to let me
trace their curlicues. I shall dust the lustrous dark mahogany coat
of the clock with my nose feather. I shall sweep away the fine bits
of dust that have settled there. I like this clock. It has its history.
Right now I imagine it would like the company of a petunia that
I will go find in the garden.

I recall a dream from some unplaceable time. I was driving an open-air car through rolling green hills. The road curved in graceful sweeping lines. I felt the irrepressible spirit of Toad in *Wind in The Willows*. Jaunty friends were with me. Their colorful garments waved and gestured in the breeze that swept through the clear blue sky. As we rounded a bend we were greeted by a lambent congregation of wild flowers. Stopping the car I moved from the driver's seat to look at the blossoms up close. I was especially taken with a giant glowing red tulip that grew fresh and stalwart from the rich dark loam. This tulip was surrounded by its compatriots — blooming avidly in all the colors of the rainbow. Lemon-yellow cups leaped up with stamen eyes of dark gold. A herd of turquoise daisies flowed up the hillside. Orange roses tangled together laughing and sensual in the hollows. Violet eyes glinted up at us from the grasses. My friends and I sniffed the fragrances that wafted into our dreaming senses. We were filled with tranquil joy.

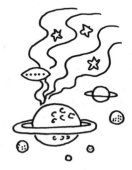

With eyes closed imagine you are standing on a green grass-covered hillside near the ocean. You reach down into the fresh grasses and pluck a dandelion. You bring the flower closer to you and note its shape and glowing color.

You take in a breath of crisp ocean air and let your attention slide down the hill to the beige sandy beach. There is a clump of driftwood sculpted into baroque shapes reminiscent of sea serpents. You savor the liquid quality of the ocean: first whispering waves on the sand, then a band of turquoise far out. Farther away you see a layer of navy blue merging into a silver line at the horizon. In the distance tiny sailboats sprout, slowly gliding out of view beyond the waves.

The sailboats twinkle whitely in your mind. They speak to you of holidays and ocean breezes on your cheeks. You are able to see one of those sailboats as clearly as if it were in your hand, or in your bath. Settle into this place that you both remember and imagine. Yawning fully in the salty air, you begin to expand. You are able to feel yourself. Your perception increases. Now you see the moon glowing silver in the pale blue sky. A round smoothness in which you can trace craters, seas and mountains.

With inspiring deep-breathing you expand once again to solar size. The nine planets are waltzing around the sun. In the background stars are laughing in the giant black velvet cushion of space. The galaxies spin and spiral gaily. They circle your mind then twirl away to vibrate dimly at the dusty edges of the universe. Ah, there, to your left, a nova celebrates its demise in red and green fireworks that splash across the light-years. Away off to your right you see a tiny black hole sipping up all its neighboring stars. Are they happy to go? In a rush they hurry to their de-enlightenment.

Coming back towards your own center you re-enter the area of Sol. There's Mars, red and striated. Venus rises green as grass. Saturn rings merrily and Pluto prowls the edges of the dance, dark and hermetic. The planets you may visit again whenever you wish. And the sun you will come back to daily. Now come back to the ocean and the tide of ground that supports you as you say 'see you soon', to the moon and to the dandelion which is draped over your knee. Remain in the internal feeling of spaciousness as you bring your attention back to your physical space. You have experienced that vision lives in you. This vision lives in your imagination, in your visual system and is accessible to you at any time. Allow this inner sense of vision to flow into the world as you open your eyes softly.

ADVANCED PRETEND: IMAGERY VARIATIONS

To gain a fresh perspective and to appreciate the experiences of other forms of being, imagine yourself *transforming* into other manifestations of nature.

Palming, imagine you are a large grey boulder residing in a high mountain meadow. You are solid all the way through. You are content to be made of quartz and mica. You carry within you tiny intriguing fossils of which you are very proud. There is a trilobite fossil barely discernible close to your top surface. When the rains come and turn your greyness to dark slate, the trilobite stands out in chalky whiteness. You sit in your rocky solidarity and the pitter-patter of rain drops on your surface. When the west wind sweeps the thick clouds away, you smile up at the yellow sun. The light heats up the mineral molecules of your skin and you glow contentedly all day. Sometimes an agile brown chipmunk with white stripes on its soft furry back comes to visit, bringing an acorn. The chipmunk tickles you as it scampers up your side. It sits serenely on your frontal prominence munching its woody brown nut.

Sometimes you watch the golden eagle soar through the high cerulean skies, sweeping its wings through the crystal clear atmosphere. When winter comes you wear a luxurious ermine mantle of clean fluffy snow. After dozing snugly through the winter months, you are the first to feel the creak and crackling of spring thaw as it subtly warms the frozen winter blankets. Sometimes you meditate on your history. Moving back in geological time, you see the era when you were a young rock under water. A dashing youthful river flowed over you from an inland sea that was teeming with flamboyantly evolving creatures. That's when you acquired your trilobite. It sank one day to rest on you and decided you would be an excellent companion through the coming eons.

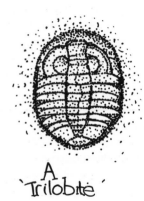

A Trilobite

Sketch a scene from the outside. Then step into it becoming a person in that setting. Use the times and places that interest you. You can become, for example, a travelling merchant in the times of Marco Polo. A cave dweller gathering roots. A pearl-diver in Japan. A runner in Peru. An Indian ...

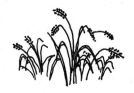

My name is Sis-Kai-Watch-Ti. I am paddling my birch bark canoe across wide bountiful marshlands. The paddle in my hands is smooth and strong. Many years ago my grandfather sat in the evening hours before the fire and carved the head of the fierce hawk on the top of my paddle. Today it dips happily in the sparkling water. I'm travelling toward the broad expanses of summer-ripened rice. The dark brown kernels fall like heavy rain into my reed baskets. A rainbow fish arches in the sun and splashes into the pale green water. I am called by the wild geese flying overhead. Their V-formation tells me that the North Wind will soon be shooting its cold arrows through the pine trees. For now the sky is warm and smells of crackling leaves and smoking campfires. The world sings its autumn song to my eyes and ears and nose.

Imagine you become a plant. A lake. A cloud. A color. A small glowing insect . . .

I'm tiny and light, spry and gleeful. When the big lantern in the sky rolls away, I come out to play. Glowing with my own joy I pirouette in the dim thickets. I dance with my friends who flicker and spin in the cool night air. We ride and glide on the night breezes. Luminous and gay, we light up our own lives with surety and merriment.

Every time you return from a transformation journey, be sure to stretch and *yawn*. And *ground* yourself.

GETTING OUT THE BUGS

When I first began to improve my own vision, I discovered in myself a terrible reluctance to imagine anything. I was in the habit of thinking my way through life. Even though I'd always had vivid dreams, I labelled myself as a non-creative, non-artistic, congested intellectual. I had started out life eager to learn, but was always tight and depressed in school settings. I could recall exactly the moment, at age twelve, when I decided to thoroughly turn off my imagery ability. I had closed my eyes one day and been completely spooked out by the images I saw. I made a firm decision never to do that again.

When it came time, at age twenty-seven, to turn my vision on and get out of the heavy myopic glasses I wore, I found my visual field in a state of desertion. My internal movie producer had long since resigned. I realized that I had to do something about the situation. One evening I sat myself down on the bathroom floor (the quietest, most protected place in the house), and asked for my imagination to re-present itself. For two or three hours I sat and watched grade D surrealistic chaos unreel before my inner eyes. My conscious mind kept running off. I had to grab it by the collar and make it sit there and watch it through.

Finally there came a time when the images calmed down. I was able to request a serene simple image and received one. Today I'm extremely grateful for the gorgeous colorful images that come to me with eyes closed or open. From these experiences, and from teaching hundreds of vision students, I know that sometimes it is necessary to transform our blocks to imaging, and to the desire to image. The following activities have been created to help dissolve these blocks. They may also provide some entertainment, polish mental skills and reactivate your brain circuits.

Suppressed negative images tend to pop up at odd, and often inconvenient, moments. They will do this until you pay them the attention they're asking for. Once you have taken a good look at and transformed them, they may benefit rather than 'bug' you.

The negative or 'spooky' images can also arise when you are relaxing. As the prevalent chatter of the verbal tape recorder in your head quiets, the unresolved negatives think they have a prime time opportunity to come in and startle you. At this point, some people will internally switch off, retreat with their awareness so that the inner vision blurs up just like physical vision does. You have the option to relate to the demons rather than retreat. Relate to them with your imagery power. This is where they get all their energy from anyway.

WHAT'S NEXT?

Take some special time for this game. Play it with a friend if possible, someone who can keep asking you 'What happens next?'

Close your eyes and ask for the scariest most unpleasant image possible to arise from your mind. You are ready now to look at this image. You know that you are the producer, director and stage manager of your internal movies. This sinister image could be a recurring anxiety picture about someone or something in your life. You might as well let it emerge now when it's under your control and transform it. If you are picking up negative images from sources other than your own mind, it's time to learn that you can edit out those pictures. We'll do this in a while with the butterfly net. In the meantime the following game is to deal with your own menacing images.

Breathing steadily and deeply, sketch and paint the spooky image in all its horrific detail. Once this is done, you or your friend ask the question, 'What happens next?'

Observe the image changes and describe them without editing. Whenever the picture gets stuck, ask the question 'What happens next?'

Continue this way, allowing the inherent healing power of your imagination to catalyze the spooky image into a state of harmlessness — until you are satisfied that the nightmare has been transformed. Once this is done, the energy tied up in that image will be freely available for you to use in positive ways.

What's the most awful thing you can imagine?

'I'm floating on my back in a lovely lagoon, relaxing in the sun. A shadow appears at the edges of my awareness. As I turn to see what's approaching, I find myself being chomped in half by a giant white shark.'

'What happens next?'

'The water gets very bloody. I see my legs sinking to the bottom of the ocean without me.'

'What happens next?'

'The shark swallows the rest of me. Everything gets very dark.'

'Yes. And then?'

'I feel myself turning into the shark.'

'How do you feel now?'

'I'm very large and sleek. I'm calm and confident. I like the deep waters. I enjoy eating.'

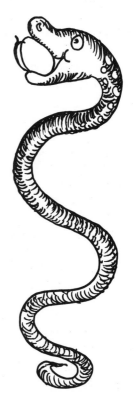

Sometimes it is helpful to enlist the aid of an ALLY.

'What's frightening you?'

'The thought of my child being kidnapped and hurt. Travis hasn't come home from school and dismissal was four hours ago. We've called all his friends. No one knows where he is.'

'What can you do beside sit and suffer?'

'I can imagine the whole neighborhood being saturated with positive protective white light.'

'What else can you imagine?'

'I can also call out an invincible wise friend to find Travis and bring him home. A kind of ally that no-one would mess with.'

'What could this be?'

'A giant black snake as big as the sidewalk. It's ancient and clairvoyant. This is my ally. I'm asking my ally to scan the neighborhood for Travis and bring him home. Ah yes, now it has found him. It is carrying Travis in an egg in its mouth. I see its long huge body sliding this way. It puts the egg gently on the doorstep and Travis steps out. Excuse me, I hear the doorbell ringing.'

Improving Vision with Imagery

ORGANIC THOUGHT EDITING

Many people say that they have trouble sitting quietly and visualizing because of persistent thoughts and ideas that keep repeating in their heads. This repetitive droning is an indication that your mental energy is travelling mainly through your left verbal brain. It is important to find a way to nudge some of this energy back into your right hemisphere or picture brain. Do this by imaging. Verbal thoughts are like butterflies or horseflies — as the case may be. Imagine yourself a horsefly net or flytrap to capture any nuisance thoughts.

Capture that thought! You've got it? Good. Now what do you do with it? You have many options. You could send it back from whence it came. You could put it in a thought-crushing machine to make thought compost. You could love and embrace it until it drops its urge to bug you. If you want to deal with it at a more convenient time, you could drop it into a lovely hand-carved filing cabinet that automatically emits thoughts at the right moment for perusal and decision.

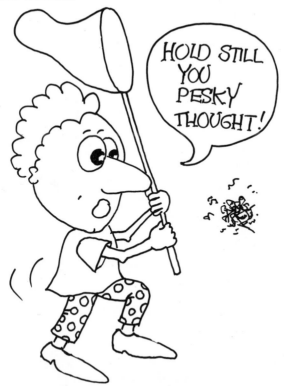

It is important that you do not identify with negative thoughts or images. Sensitive people often pick up the output from other people's minds without realizing it. If this is happening with you, do some mental housecleaning.

A vision student once told me that every time he palmed his eyes and imagined a beautiful ocean beach he had to deal with the sight of litter and pollution. Oil slicks smeared the turquoise waters, empty beer cans and paper wrappers befouled the white sands. No matter how he tried to visualize something pleasant, old negative associations interfered.

Rather than let the litter lie in his visual field, we went into imagery clean-up action. This student sketched for himself a huge vacuum cleaner. He diligently slurped up all the debris on the ocean and land with his super-duper debris scooper. Therefore each time garbage appeared in his images, he immediately cleaned it up. Eventually the garbage got tired of this treatment and stopped coming around. These solutions are suggestions. Devise your own imaginative solutions for taking care of your inner visions.

Another reluctance some people experience has to do with fear of the darkness. Taking your mind into pleasant darkness journeys may ease away this anxiety. It will also help your mind and eyes relax for night-time seeing.

TRAVELS IN THE DARK

Sit or *lie down* in a quiet place. *Close* your eyes. *Imagine* that you are camping in the countryside at night. Your sleeping bag is ebony canvas lined with dark, rich silk. It is filled with the down of black swans. As you look up into the sky, you see tiny diamond stars scattered across the infinite nothingness of space. Your attention is called back to the darkened earth by a freshening breeze that glides towards you through the shadowed trees. The scent of rain enters your nostrils. A large black cloud moves over you obscuring all the stars. Soon you are enveloped in silent blackness. You feel the coolness of the cloud, but you know if it decides to empty itself of its watery burden, the wetness will simply slide off your physical body while refreshing your mental processes. Scan around you with the feather of a crow. Caress the deep inky shadows. Let your body melt into the darkness. Feel secure and content in your dark night nest. You hear the double call of an owl. You smell the plants as they quiver in anticipation of the coming rain. Gems of moisture touch your cheek. Time to snuggle deep into your warm cocoon. You are falling asleep in the soft shadows, resting profoundly until the first rays of morning sunlight spill over your eyelids.

THE 'TOO BUSY' GAME

'I don't have time to sit and visualize because I am *too busy*'. 'This stuff is great but I have no time for it.' If you are enamoured of busyness or are convinced that it is necessary to existence, I have good news for you. You don't have to give it up to incorporate vision

and imagery in your life. What you do is *integrate* visualization
into your usual tasks. If, for example, you have decisions to make
or problems to resolve, make your creative imagery a part of the
process.

You want to make:

    a business decision
    a family decision
    a financial determination
    a change in your behavior
    study for exams
    learn a new skill

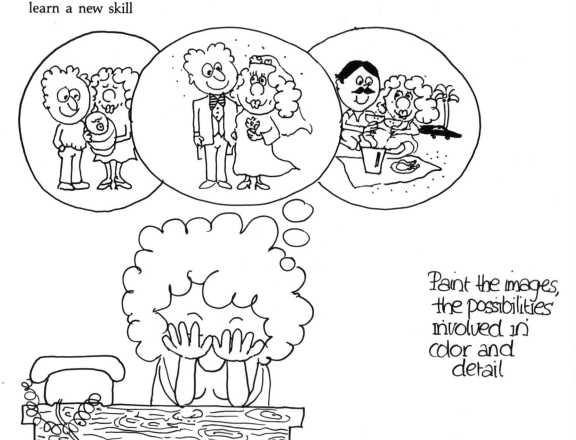

Paint the images, the possibilities involved in color and detail

    Sit or *lie down, palm* your eyes, and *ask* for all the factors in
the situation to appear. *Paint* the images, the possibilities involved
in color and detail. Visualize the possible variations of the solution
as trails into a forest. Each trail ends in a meadow. Each meadow
is home to a single possible solution. Travel to one meadow and
explore, savor, study that one solution. When you have satisfied
yourself with that one possibility walk back to your original starting point and take the forest path to another meadow. Visit the

variation there. Act it out with costumes and props. When finished with investigating this possibility, return again to the starting point. Take as many trips down the paths to the meadows as needed. Keep the solutions separated by the forest. When you return finally to the starting place you may make your final decision based on the satisfied feeling that came from visualizing one of the possible solutions. You will have integrated seeing and thinking. You will have blended the power of imagination and intuition with your analytical abilities.

Chapter 8

Improving Vision with Sun, Light, and Color

We are children of the solar system. Our human eyes were shaped in the effulgence of the sun. As diurnal creatures we see best in clear daylight. The more we deprive our eyes of natural light by constant indoor living the more our eyes lose this ability to respond visually. Every day we wake up. Every day we are meant to have light. In fact, our whole endocrine system is attuned to the pulse of the sun's spectrum. The colors of the rainbow sing various songs to our being by affecting the hypothalamus, a brain area that regulates emotions, pupil size and accommodation. Ultraviolet light streaming into the eyes, when uninhibited by window or eyeglasses, rouses the pituitary gland, the concert master of the glands that secrete hormones regulating growth, metabolism, assimilation and sexual expression. For more exciting information about the effect of sunlight on your body and endocrine system, read John Ott's book *Health and Light*, and Zane Kime, M.D. *Sunlight Can Save Your Life*.

The drastic increase in visual imbalances in populations has coincided with the move from rural to urban life. The conveniences of urbanized technology have brought with them the disrupting effects of fluorescent lighting, video display units, and sedentary lifestyles in enclosed static rooms. It is up to us to re-orient ourselves to the sun, the source and medium of our ability to see. Our physical, mental and creative selves will flourish and grow rather than decline and dim. Clarity, glow and sparkle return to eyes once they come out of the stuffy rooms to play in the luminosity of the generous sun.

We accomplish this return to the sun by integrating the Sunning Games into our work, play, sport and daily duties.

THE SUNNING GAME

Place yourself comfortably facing the sun. *Close your eyes.*

Begin to draw a counterclockwise circle with your nose. Continue this movement as you open up your mind to the sun's warmth and energy.

Natural Vision Improvement

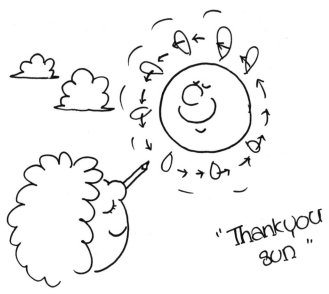

"Thankyou sun"

As you circle, say thank you to the sun for its generous gift of light, color and warmth.

Imagine the large globe in the sky is a sunflower. *Trace* a smooth circle on the sunflower with your nose. As you circle the flower, its petals may seem to revolve in the opposite direction of your movement. Your action and the rhythmic image of the petals will induce fine saccadic movements while the light enters the opening doors of your mind. *Ask* the sunlight to flow deeply into the farthest reaches of your psyche. *Cleanse* the inside of your visual field with clear white liquid light. Let it sweep through all the nooks and crannies to renew and refresh your being. When your mind is cleared, trace down the stalk of your sunflower to its roots in the earth.

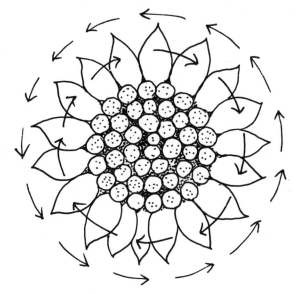

Improving Vision with Sun,
Light, and Color

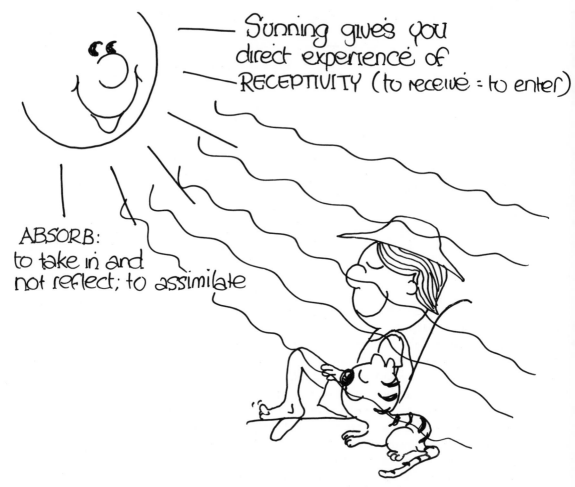

Sunning gives you direct experience of RECEPTIVITY (to receive = to enter)

ABSORB:
to take in and not reflect; to assimilate

Visualize a picket fence in front of you. The fence is white as is the feather you now place on your nose. The fence extends to infinity to the right and left of you.

With your nose feather tickle the fence from side to side. As you travel left the fence slides to the right. Keep doing this action until you feel a sense of release in your mind and eyes. If your blur is in the distance begin with imaging your picket fence close in front of you at a distance you can imagine easily (1 to 3 feet). After feathering the fence at this distance imagine that it moves farther away from you. You can end up with your fence in the far distance. It can be tiny or large.

If your blur is up close proceed in the opposite order. Begin with the image of the picket fence far away. Gradually bring your fence in closer and closer until it is within 3 inches of your nose and tiny — the fence around a doll house.

Feel free to vary the color and distances of any of these images to suit yourself. Do not get stuck in always visualizing at one distance.

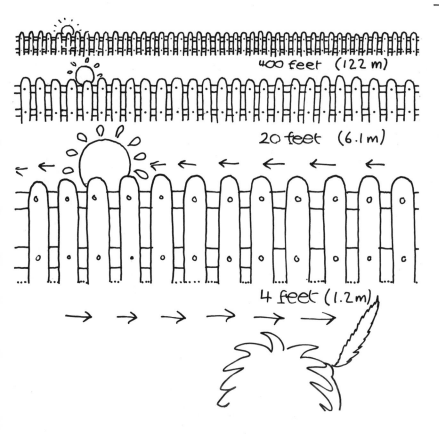

400 feet (122 m)

20 feet (6.1 m)

4 feet (1.2 m)

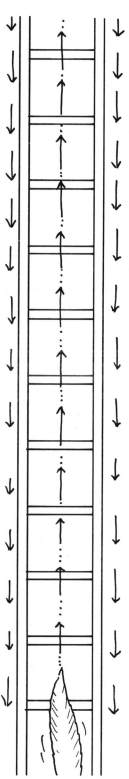

Remember to move toward flexibility. Also start out these games by imaging where it is easy and carry that ease into other areas. This is why near-sighted people start with images close and move them outward. The opposite is true for far-sighted folk. If you have blur at all distances then play the game at all distances.

Imagine there is a tall ladder in front of the sun that extends into the heavens and deep into the earth. With your nose feather slide up and down the rungs of the ladder. As you move down, let the ladder slide up. As you go upward, the ladder slips down. Vary the distance of the ladder from you as you did the picket fence. All this time your eyes are closed. Stretch and yawn at any point. The more, the better.

The above activities open up your vision to the light and produce saccadic motions in all directions. Horizontal, vertical and circular.

PLAYING IN THE RAINBOW

Out of the 'white' light of the sun comes all the colors of the rainbow. Each color speaks to a certain part of our body. Color communicates to our subconscious mind. We may ask colors to help us in many areas. The following color code and examples will provide

Improving Vision with Sun, Light, and Color

you with material to integrate creativity into your life. While sunning or palming use the following ideas as springboards to relating with the rainbow colours.

RED is the color which invigorates and strengthens the physical body. 'I am sunning and asking for the red ray of the sun to enter every cell in my body. This ruby light is giving me physical vigor and energy. My red blood cells travel through my body with extra vitality. All my muscles and organs are being strengthened. Red is warmth, congeniality, sexuality. I am being cloaked in a crimson light. I soak it in until a healthy glow blooms through my skin. I have the jauntiness of the red cardinal, the elegance of the scarlet rose, the glory of a blazing sunset.'

ORANGE is the emotional energy. It is the bridge between the physical and the mental, and the central axis of 3-dimensional perception. The stronger the emotions, the more powerful a person can be. The question is, can one handle the emotion without its being destructive to body or environment?

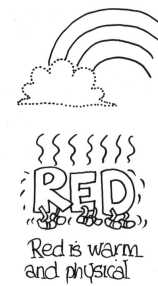

Red is warm and physical

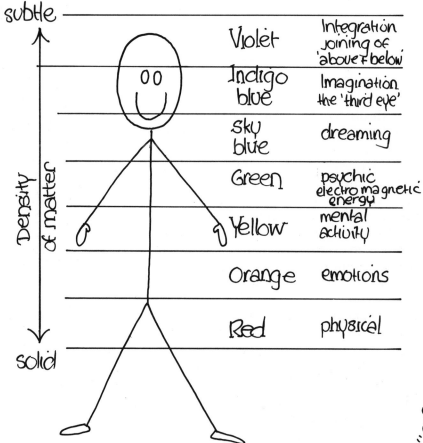

Violet	Integration joining of 'above + below'
Indigo blue	Imagination the 'third eye'
Sky blue	dreaming
Green	psychic electromagnetic energy
Yellow	mental activity
Orange	emotions
Red	physical

subtle

Density of matter

solid

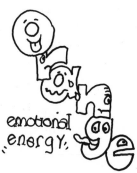

emotional energy

Palm your eyes. *Imagine* that you are striding through a field of brilliant orange poppies abrim with sunlight. As you stride through the nodding blossoms they touch you gently and your garments turn to orange. Topping the rise of the hill, you look down into a cupped valley that glows like a tangerine skin turned inside out. In this valley a small tree grows plush with velvety orange apricots. A pumpkin-colored horse is eating the apricots off the tree. Its topaz mane ripples in the sunlight. Momentarily startled by your presence, the horse snorts and wheels around to assess you with its yellow sapphire eyes. Pausing, you calmly breathe in the aromatic air and open your mind to the spirit of this glowing creature. A voice begins to speak inside your head and you listen carefully. 'I am the wild spirit of your emotions. My spirit is the golden fire that glows in the centre of your body. I live my life attuned to the flow and swirl of colors around you. I hear music and dance with your body. I rise up and run with the wild winds. There are times when the wintry season overtakes me. The rivers at which I drink are frozen over, the heavy snows slow me down. Still my fiery spirit glows unnoticed, banked under the layers of muffling stillness — a slow heavy season. When spring comes I respond with verve, leaving the past behind. You may think that at times I am afraid when wolves howl or the earth shakes. Yet even at these times my strong spirit rides the waves and brings me back to this place of golden tranquility where I munch the juicy apricots and saucily prance through the wild orange poppies'.

YELLOW is the color that represents conscious mental thought, which could be a glorious lucid function of the human experience. It relates to the solar plexus. Meditating with yellow may soothe your tummy. While sitting in the sun or in your room turn your mind to yellow, the wavelength that produces the sensations of lemons and daffodils.

Let the yellow wave sing into your mind. It takes your intellect for a journey. You walk down a path paved with yellow bricks to a wall that stretches high to the right and to the left. The wall looks solid and impassable. You see writing on the wall in bright yellow paint. Letters that flow into words. The words tickle your mind as they did when you first learned to read. The words lead you to the right, gradually forming themselves into sentences. 'This wall is an illusion' you read. 'Thoughts are whatever you want them to be — masters, servants, playmates, friends or enemies. Thoughts come and go at your command.' As you move along the wall, imagine touching it with your hand. You find the wall becoming softer, the hardness of it is gradually changing to a liquid consistency that your hand breaks through. With both hands now push the wall aside and step through it with your whole body. Looking around you see several smiling ladies seated in classical poses. The first

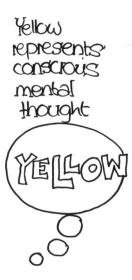

Improving Vision with Sun, Light, and Color

lady is dressed in saffron silk and a wreath of small golden flowers encircles her dark brown hair. She is holding a book that she extends to you. Taking up the book you notice to your surprise that it weighs very little in spite of its large volume. It is covered with gold leaf and a single circle is inscribed on the front. Opening the book you see geometric forms that appear to dance and move about like an old folk dance. 'What does this mean?' you enquire of the woman. 'This book shows you the patterns of your thinking mind', she replies. 'The patterns that are basic to your mind are shown to you without specific content. By absorbing the images of this book you will see that you are able to think clearly at all times. You will be able to connect and rearrange thoughts, picking and choosing the thoughts you wish to use to form and influence your life. Take the book with you. I wish you joy as you play with your intelligence.' The lady then disappears as do her companions who will reappear upon your next visit into the yellow world. The atmosphere around you becomes suffused with a golden glow. Your mind is bathed in clear yellow, a thought-less state that prepares you for a new return to thinking and communicating in your daily life.

GREEN represents the electromagnetic energy. The yellow in the green is the connection between the electromagnetic mind and the physical organic brain. The green actually attracts information according to the brain's ability to assimilate and coordinate it.

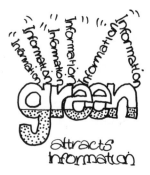

Someday when you are sunning (or palming) take the following adventure:

Imagine that you are walking down a forest pathway lined with stately spruce trees. The path is laced with the trailing fronds of graceful ferns. Underfoot a thick carpet of moss cushions your steps. You see fastened to the trunk of a noble spruce a green sign. Painted on this sign (which you are outlining with your nose pencil of course) are white words which say 'This Way To The Emerald Lady'. You proceed to the front door of a small cottage completely covered with dark green ivy. You knock on the carved jade door. It opens and a cool voice says, 'Come in'. You enter a sea green room where the sunlight spills through a skylight on to a tiny woman clothed from head to toe in bayberry leaves. On her head is a Peter Pan cap sporting a dashing green feather. You feel welcome, loved and cherished in this room. The petite green lady brings you to a table of malachite to show you a deck of cards in the shape of fig leaves. She tosses the cards up in a swirling shower. One card descends in front of you. You decide what the image on the card is. Developing clear and vivid green will enable your imagined pictures to become physical realities.

BLUE is the dream vibration. Its strength determines one's ability to exist within inner worlds while maintaining a physical body.

Your dreams are the first level of experience that is completely non-technical.

Ask that the blue frequency of the sunlight distribute itself throughout your body and mind. The sensation of the blue is cool and subtle within you. Dress yourself in a bathing costume the color of a summer sky. Walk across the evening sand toward the water.

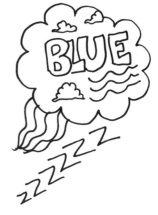

Blue is the dream vibration

Spread your arms wide at the ocean's edge and inhale the tangy air. Feel the *warm* breeze caress your skin as it floats over the sun-heated sand. The setting sun shines from its reddish disc, a sinking eye in the west. Its light shows you a wavering orange blade laid on the soft blue sea. You walk into the waters. Step in deeper until the blue surrounds you. Close your eyes again and acknowledge that you are immersed in the universe of blue. This is the corridor that leads you into dreams. The blue takes you into the place where your subtler minds speak and create holograms called dreams. Pause here in the doorway, breathe and know that you exist completely solid and self-aware in the blue corridor. The waters may wash over you and give you momentary anxiety, yet you know that your body began in these swirling, living waters. Your dreaming confidence is undaunted. The blue is your friend. You know that the limitless sky and your limited dreaming are linked. Inhale the blue color again and ask that your mind and body be soothed and calmed in the gentleness of pervasive sky blue.

INDIGO. Red comes into the blue to create indigo, combining the physical with the higher mental abilities. Indigo is the true seeing level, the vibration of the imagination.

You are sitting in the sun. Imagine that you arise and walk into a large open kitchen. All the walls are white as are the floor and ceiling. On the white stove is an enormous white enamel pot. Standing over the pot with a long wooden ladle in her hand is a young woman. As you enter the light-filled kitchen she lifts her head and with a smile invites you to glance inside the pot. There you see a deep wine-colored liquid boiling, spurting tiny droplets of color combining deep blue with red. 'This is the color of imagination', the young woman states as she carefully lowers a large white cloth into the bubbling cauldron. 'We'll stir this for a few moments then you can help me take the cloth out into the sunlight to dry.'

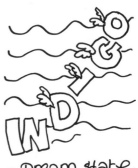

- Dream state

She lifts the dripping burgundy cloth into the watertight basket you hold. You take it outdoors and spread the cloth over four poles. A tent-like structure is created. When the sunlight shines through you are irresistibly drawn to sit under the canopy of indigo cloth. It's like walking into a cool soup of plum-colored light. Perhaps a few drops of dye fall on your head, no matter: you sit and let the indigo light filter into your body and mind. You breathe steadily and imagine the right side of your brain and the left side of your brain flooding with indigo, the red and the blue colors combining to create a dreamlike ability in the physical world. Imagination and creativity are your subconscious legacy. This color will open the treasure chest. Who knows what may happen now? As you sit in the indigo light, visualize a coruscating glow appearing at your forehead. Feel the energy of your resourceful mind coming forward to shine through your smooth and peaceful brow. Be content in this color, non-directive, serene, aware.

VIOLET. More red and more blue allows one to bring the power of all the colors into physical reality.

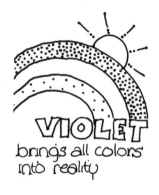

VIOLET
brings all colors into reality

Imagine that you are sitting on a violet carpet. The stuff of the carpet is thick and soft to your touch. It glows in the sunlight, the color that inhabits amethysts and lavender flowers. Imagine that a turban of violet light is wound around the top of your head. Turbaned and carpeted you lift off into the air to take a ride into a purple sunset. Everything you need you have. Everything you could be, you are becoming. The violet carpet can take you anywhere you want to go, physically, mentally, spiritually. The violet symbolizes the blending and integration of all the various aspects of yourself. Riding along on a mountainside breeze you see purple asters smiling up at you from a grassy meadow. Your purple carpet lifts you over a craggy peak that is enshrouded in a violet mist. It carries you over a chasm whose throat is purple-black and brings you to rest before a giant crystal ball. You step off the carpet and walk over to the ball which is taller than your head. The ball's surface is a mirror. You see yourself in violet reflection in the ball. Especially you notice your eyes smiling back at you, brightly gleaming, clearly seeing.

INDOOR LIGHTING

The best light for all visual purposes is direct sunlight being received by relaxed mobile eyes in a healthy body. The next best source of illumination under artifical conditions is incandescent lighting. It has been shown that fluorescent light can cause eyestrain and produce myopia. Through muscle testing it has been demonstrated that fluorescent oscillation tends to short circuit the flow of brain energy. If you *have* to work in an office under fluorescent lights, bring in your own incandescent desk fixture to shine on your paper work. *Sun* your eyes at lunch hour. Balance stressful tasks such as working with VDUs in air-conditioned, noisy, fluorescent-flooded offices by sunning, palming, breathing and yawning for short periods each day.

At home, shine as much as 150 watts on your immediate visual activity and turn off unnecessary lights in the rest of the house. Your eyes and mind love the contrast that high illumination pro-

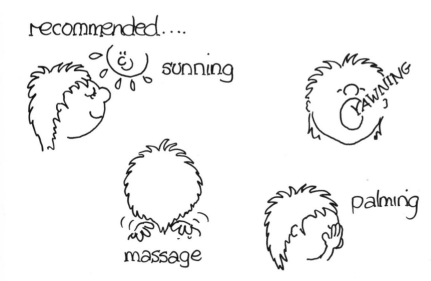

recommended....

sunning

yawning

massage

palming

vides. Once your eyes are completely relaxed in all circumstances you will be able to function in dimmer surroundings.

APPROPRIATE SUNNING

The sunlight invigorates every part of your retina. There is no need to open the eyes in the sun. Adequate warmth and energy will move through your closed eyelids and there is no chance of sunburning your retina — a subject which causes great consternation among some eye doctors who can be heard admonishing 'And don't *ever* stare into the sun.' As a natural vision student you won't be staring anywhere, let alone into the sun. Keeping your eyes closed, gently and smoothly moving your whole head while sunning ensures relaxation while you absorb the beneficial healing rays of the sun.

I suggest that you sun for five to ten minutes each day when the sun is at a convenient angle, usually in the morning or afternoon. If it is winter and the sun is low, sun any time during the day. If you find yourself sitting outdoors only on the weekends then incorporate *sun-dipping* into your work-a-day life.

As you walk from work to the parking lot, pause for a moment, *close your eyes* and make a short smooth circlet around the sun. Open your eyes and proceed. Even a few seconds of sunning integrated here and there during the day will benefit you far more than rushing headlong and head down from business to task to duty to errand to fatigue. Greet the sun as you would a dear friend on the street, momentarily but thoroughly.

Become empty-headed, simple-minded. It's a relief after thinking and connecting and solving all day long. On the heart level you are experiencing the giving, generosity and warmth of the

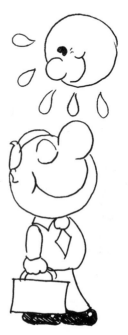

Improving Vision with Sun, Light, and Color

sun. All descriptions of heart and heartiness. The sun loves us all equally. The sun will cleanse.

Sun the ears and throat, and soles of the feet as well.

SPECIAL CONSIDERATIONS

1. The retina of the eye is delicate. The sun can burn holes in its membrane so keep your eyes closed. Prevent sunburn. Our skin takes six months to completely recover from sunburn. Build your capacity for light slowly but surely.

2. If need be the pinhole spectacles can be used in an extreme situation of lots of light that you're not prepared for — such as a first weekend on a sailboat. After a few months of sunning, even students who were skiers reported that the glare off the snow was reduced to the point where they could enjoy their weekend on the slopes without using sunglasses. Also the glass of cheaper sunglasses can have unnoticed warps which cause the eyes to strain looking through the lenses. The colors in the lenses may have a deleterious effect on the autonomic body systems, and the healthy ultraviolet light is blocked out. The wearing of sunglasses does not alter the conceptual fear and incapacity for light. It perpetuates the weakness.

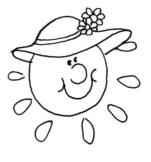

wear a hat

3. If you find in the beginning that the sunlight is too strong for you, start out in the shade of a tree. Our approach is to ease into things, to do the minimum and feel secure and pleasant at every step. The *sunning* activity can actually be done anywhere, even in a darkened room where you imagine the sun. If the weather is grey and foggy, use a simple light source such as a regular incandescent light bulb or an infra-red heat lamp. *Never* use an ultraviolet suntanning lamp to sun your eyes. These artificial ultraviolet bulbs do not give you the warning of *too much heat* that the sun gives you when you've over-exposed your winter body to summer sun.

4. If you have very sensitive skin, apply some cream to your face and be sure the sun is low when you spend your five minutes absorbing the light.

5. If you are not overly sensitive to the sun spend as much time sunning as you like, using commonsense to protect your skin.

After *sunning*, you may wish to practice *sketching* or other vision activities in this book. For this you will turn around with your back to the sun. The sunlight will then illuminate your reading material, your photograph (as in the painting game, page 99) or the environment in front of you.

THE TWELVE SOLAR BENEFITS

After a few months of some amount of regular *sunning*, you will
find that:

1. Your light tolerance will have expanded. No more frowns,
   wrinkles and squinting in the bright light of the day.
2. You may experience *flashes* of clarity after a bit of sunning
   as colors take on intensity and details begin to jump out
   at you.
3. The appearance of your eyes becomes healthy and attractive. No more need to hide yellowish, bleary eyes behind
   'shades'. The eyes of students who love their sunning blaze
   with energy and sparkle.
4. The urge to 'fight the light' and pop on sunglasses will go
   away. The increase of your light capacity eliminates glare
   and photo-sensitivity.
5. Your night perception and ability to visualize darkness will
   increase. Students have reported that during a sunning session they alternated palming with sunning. The depth of
   velvety blackness experienced was thrilling. This is a sure
   sign of deep internal relaxation.
6. The warmth of the sun relaxes tight eye muscles which then
   release their grip on the eyeball. The eyeball is let free to
   vibrate.
7. The light stimulates the retinal cells, pituitary gland and
   the visual cortex.
8. The movement you make while sketching the images
   encourages rapid saccadic vibrations.
9. Your right, imagining hemisphere of the brain is turned on
   to increase visual stimulation and energy through the whole
   body.
10. You are receiving all the healing colors contained in direct
    sunlight.
11. The strong energy of stimulation to the non-physical bodies
    will bring up an excitement and thrill that result in happy
    emotional responsiveness. The sunlight is a natural force,
    free and available to everyone. The light is going to shine
    on your mental attitudes, your emotional state and your
    physical capabilities.
12. The sunlight will clear the intellectual mind, tone your
    emotional energies and feed the spiritual minds (the non-
    material aspects of yourself, your imaginations, dreams and
    connections to finer universal vibrations).

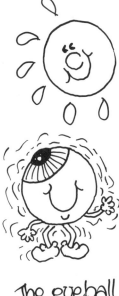

The eyeball
is let free
to vibrate

Improving Vision with Sun,
Light, and Color

Chapter 9

Improving Vision with Mandalas

The mandala is a visual form which has a powerful effect on both the conscious and unconscious minds. Its infinite variations occur throughout nature and have been utilized by artists in many cultures. The mandala concentrates energy through its circular rhythm which has no beginning and no end. It has the effect of bringing you back to yourself. The requisite property of a mandala is its centre which like the centre of our mental attention reverberates outward into space. Its shape illustrates symmetry and harmonious relationships. Its geometry, coloring and depicted forms such as animals, the sun, moon and preternatural beings symbolically reverberate through the human psyche. If you drop a pebble into a tranquil pond, you will have created a natural mandala. Pause for a moment and imagine this.

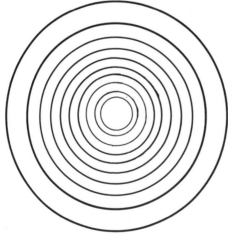

Viewing the mandala causes us to resonate with a basic pattern of life energy. It encourages us to join the little picture — the micro-

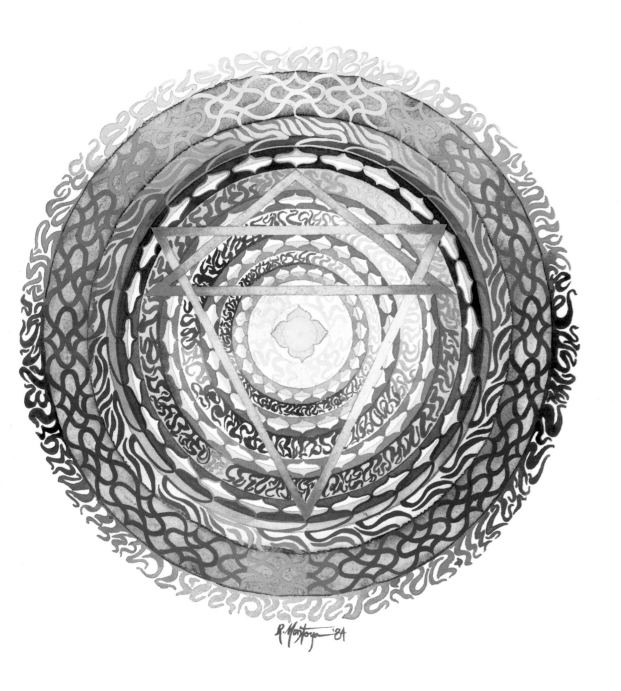

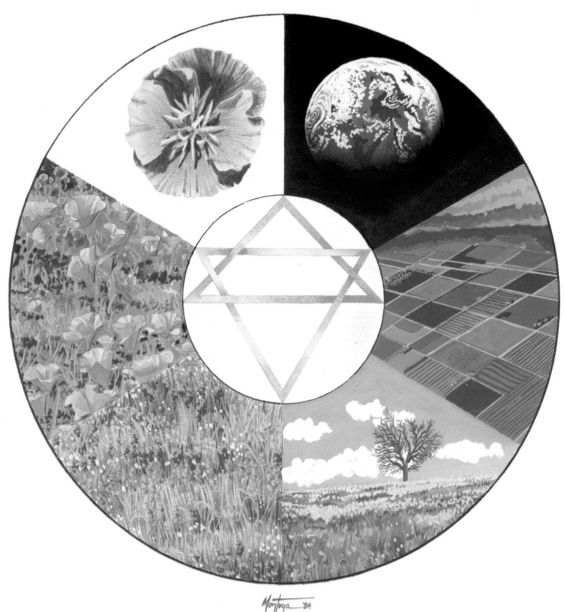

Montoya '84

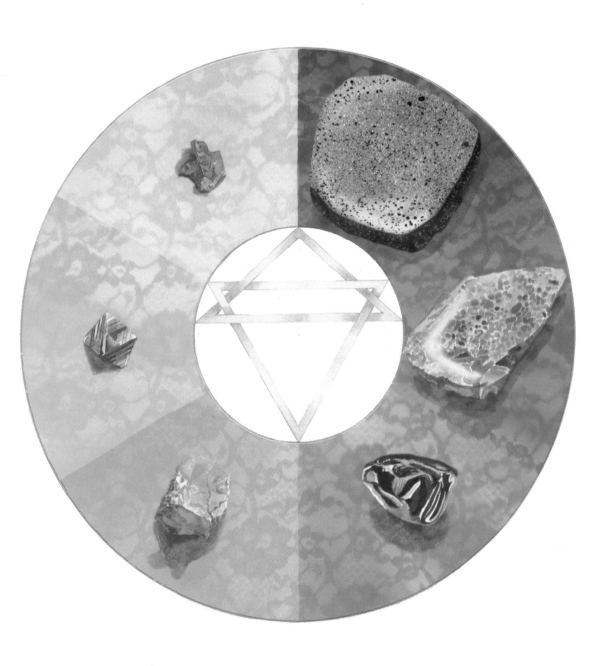

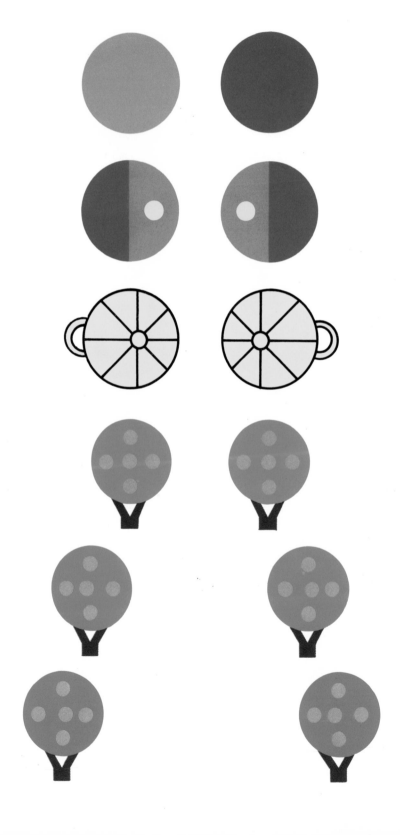

cosm, with the big picture — the macrocosm. The conscious ego-self which says, '*I see*' reaches toward the mysterious forces which swirl the planets and galaxies. The effects of spending time with mandala forms are the centering of oneself, calming of the nervous system and entering a state of peacefulness. This sensation of inner wholeness accompanies clarity of vision. It is also possible that the beauty of the mandala's inner harmonies will lift your thought patterns out of stale negative tracks on to positive attractive pathways.

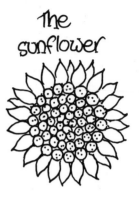

Let's find some mandalas close to us. Our mind flies to the sun, a flaming orb with an atomic heart that shines on our faces. Then to the plants that feed from the sun. Especially we note the sunflower which you've visited already. Be aware now of its mandalic effect as you edge its shape while sunning. Certainly our own eyes are mandalas. Take a look at your irises in a mirror. See the centre of the pupil which is the passageway *from the outside world to your inner theater*. Even the retina at the back of the eyes is roundish with a central concentrated area which we will explore in chapter 11.

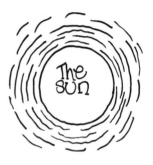

The reason for emphasizing the mandala form is to have an easy enjoyable way to stimulate the liveliness of the eyes while the mind is being soothed and centred. Eventually we want saccadic movements to occur without having to think about them. The multiple harmonious non-linear, right brain images of the mandalas invite your eyes into saccadic motion. Gazing across sparkling water, into the branches of trees or though natural crystals will do this also. With mandalas we have the added advantage of the continuous curve revolving about a point. It helps to keep the mind from wandering.

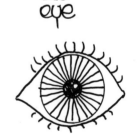

In this chapter we'll acquaint ourselves with general and special purpose mandalas. Begin with the color plates. Then move to the black and white mandalas. From there you can decide which images will be the most useful for you to carry around in your mind to activate at opportune moments.

COLOR PLATE 1: THE SACCADIC FIRE WHEEL

Hold the image at arm's length to start. Imagine your magic feather is on the end of your nose. Gently brush around the outside of the wheel moving in an anticlockwise direction, blinking nonchalantly. Slide your feather to the next inner circle. Your mind begins to mellow. Close your eyes for a few moments continuing to glide round the image in your mind! Tiny rhythmical pulses are flowing through your eyes and head. Open your eyes again and allow your attention to gradually spiral into the center toward the small and specific converging point which represents the cosmic source. Now meander idly, playing with the mandala. Its colors and shapes will amuse your attention with mellifluous visual harmonies. Close your eyes again and attend the after images that arise from the fire wheel. Allow them to expand merrily into space, enlarging the fire wheel.

If you spiral outwardly in an anticlockwise direction you will be encouraging the radiating energy of expansive expression. Conversly, moving clockwise toward the centre will gather and centre energy, a focusing of attention. Play with the images spiraling in both directions.

COLOR PLATE 2: THE MICRO-MACRO WHEEL

Designed to inspire eye mobility together with near-far accommodation, this mandala serves to move the mind and imagination beyond their usual stamping grounds.

A close start: Hold the picture at reading distance. Edge the area of the wheel where the poppy is magnified. Scan this section with your nose feather, eyes open. Imagine the smell of the delicate petals. Savor the feeling you would have when touching the flower. Close your eyes and do the same in your imagination. Open your eyes and move to the next area. Repeat the absorption of the shapes and colors from this new perspective. Close again to affirm this perspective. Then move on repeating this simple process.

Flexion: Trace and rollick about from close to far, and from far to close, on the micro-macro wheel. Close and visualize at any point of view. Bring the images to life by using all your senses. Walk into the field, hold the earth in the palm of your hand.

Continue with this cycle of eyes open, scan, eyes closed, imagine, until you arrive at the most distant point of view. Breathe broadly. Acknowledge 'I am a relaxed distance see-er.'

A far beginning: Hold the picture at reading distance. Edge the area of the wheel at the top right where our planet is serenely turning in space. Close your eyes and paint the earth in front of you. Move your nose gently from right to left across the swirling oceans and continents. Notice the earth rocking from side to side. Feel the tranquility garnered from this broad overview. Luxuriate in this sensation and bring it to the next area of the wheel as you open your eyes. Scan the next closer view. Repeat this process. Contemplate the feelings and your ability to relate softly to images as they draw closer and closer to you. End up with the face of the poppy a few inches from your nose. Acknowledge, 'I am a relaxed close see-er.'

COLOR PLATE 3: GLOWING GEMS: FOR PRESBYOPES AND HYPEROPES

Hold the third color plate at reading distance. Starting at the upper left hand section, brush across the mineral specimen with a soft nose feather. Then close your eyes imagining that the rock has come into physical being, arising up out of the page. Your feather sweeps across the grainy texture that your mind is visualizing. The endless but specific variations of specks, glints, tiny ledges and grooves fashion themselves for you out of your past meetings with the mineral kingdom. Recall the nature of beige sand, grey shale, blue lapis lazuli and green malachite. Open your eyes once more and sweep across the painted stone with which you began. It may now appear three-dimensional, clearer, leaping off the page. Continue this same procedure around the color plate with each stone in turn.

THE WHEEL OF HEARTS: FOR ASTIGMATISM

The wheel of hearts is for smoothing out the blur that comes with astigmatism. The angle at which your eye has formed astigmatic blur can be revealed from your eyeglasses prescription. However it may need deciphering by your eye doctor or optician. The multiplication of edges experienced with astigmatism can happen at any point of the compass. For example, you might have a cylindrical lens in your glasses which correct for astigmatism at 180°.

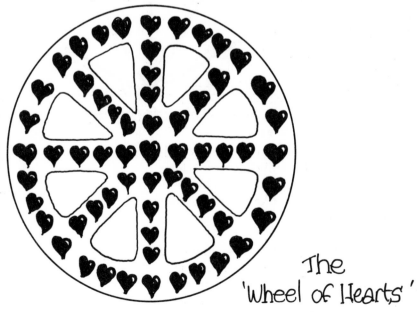

The 'Wheel of Hearts'

This means that horizontal lines are more indistinct. It is also possible to have horizontal astigmatism in one eye and oblique astigmatism
in the other eye. So for general purposes let's trace the lines of the
compass in all directions.

Hold the wheel of hearts at a comfortable distance in front of you,
circle counterclockwise around the outer rim with your fluffy nose
feather. Slide over the hearts as you go. Close your eyes and continue.
Image the shimmering hearts as you circle. Open your eyes again
and slide from side to side on the horizontal spoke of the wheel.
Close and visualize. Open and repeat this action with each spoke
of the wheel. Slip the wheel of hearts into your mental valise and
bring it out at odd moments. Put it on walls of buildings, on
windows, on a tree.

After spending some time with the wheel of hearts, which is
soft in its contours, we will want to gradually move to more specific,
sharper edges, keeping our automatic saccades prevailing all along.

Place an imaginary black felt-tipped marker on the end of your
nose and circle the *beaded fan*. Then begin to loosely sweep on
the beaded radii one by one. Your marker traces the lines. When
you close your eyes, reproduce the whole image in your mind. The
beads will stimulate saccadic movements just from your imagining
them. Visualize the beads in decorator colors if you like, vibrant
purple, apple green, plush pink, siren cerise.

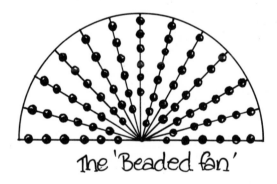

The 'Beaded fan'

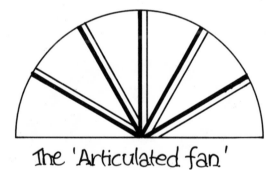

The 'Articulated fan'

Finally move to the *articulated fan* where the lines are crisp and
austere. Do the same as with the *beaded fan* only this time when
you open your eyes you will be carrying with you in the back of
your mind, the sensation, of ease and clarity. Play with this fan
to hone your ability to mentally move along straight lines — seeing
them single, brisk and decisive.

Making free with the mandala form, we shall now double it
to make the eight-track which is also the ancient sign for infinity
and for integration of the right and the left hemispheres. Begin at the
center and start counterclockwise with your little engine. Follow
the track repeatedly through its interweaving patterns. When you

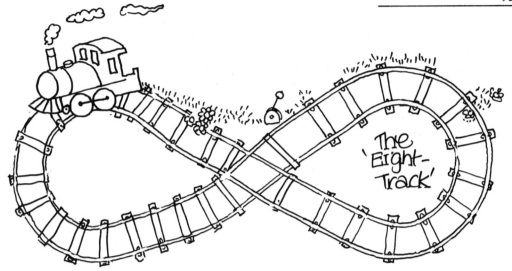

close your eyes you may bring toyfilled memories of your childhood back to color up the engine. Let flowers spring up between the ties, tow fascinating treasures behind the engine as it leads your nose around the eight-track. Needless to say, this activity you are able to take anywhere. Expand the game to flow around tree trunks. Close the eyes and move the train across continents deviating from and then returning to the circular form time and again.

THE CENTRING SPIRAL

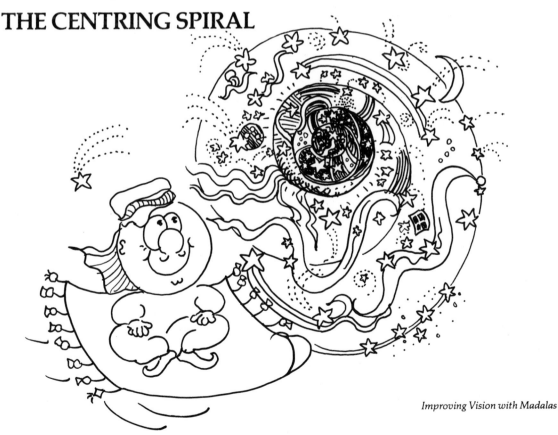

Improving Vision with Madalas

You are Ali Baba on your magic carpet. At the sound of the words, 'Open Sesame' you find yourself floating in space lifted high on your Persian rug. Before you appears a spiral of pure energy, a galaxy of stars rotating; suspended in the inky blackness of space. It seems so close you could reach up and touch the outer spiral which, as you watch, expands through, around and beyond you. The motion relaxes you, drawing your vision inwards, following the spiral ever-inwards to a centre that stretches away to the infinite. You contemplate this spiral, feeling its rhythm, hearing its song and seeing the broader dance of life.

Chapter 10

Seeing for Yourself: a First Basic Program

THE BASICS ARE FOR EVERYONE

Even the visually-balanced folks who have no need for glasses will benefit from the basic activities which serve them in a preventative or enhancing fashion. For those of us who have already stepped out of glasses, the basics become lifelong habits and ensure the ongoing harmony and clarity of our vision.

You who are enthused about bettering your sight now have an understanding of the effects of movement, light and imagery on your vision. These three areas form the foundation for launching your own program. We will now delineate which natural vision games are important for you based on whether your sight is blurry in the distance or up close. Then we will do the Painting Game which blends together all the activities learned so far in a way that results in 'flashes' of clarity.

CLEARING THE DISTANCE BLUR: FOR MYOPIA AND ASTIGMATISM

Activate 'edging' and 'sketching' all the time with your nose pencil. See chapter 6, p. 49. Sometimes you'll find yourself in a brown studious stare. That's OK. Simply take a deep breath and move on.

Develope your imagery for distance by 'palming'. Do this for at least five minutes during the day wherever you find yourself. If your eyes call out to you from fatigue or stress, palm and visualize to rest them. See chapter 7, p. 63.

Invest in a bit of sunning whenever you are able. See chapter 8, p. 78. Sit down and relax for at least five minutes. If not that, do a little sundipping on the way to the car, while waiting for the street light to change, or hanging out the clothes. See p. 87.

Utilize the mandala images at times, particularly the ones which take you into the distance, flexing your ability to fluidly move

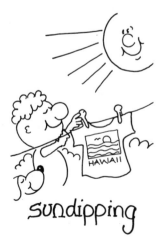

sundipping

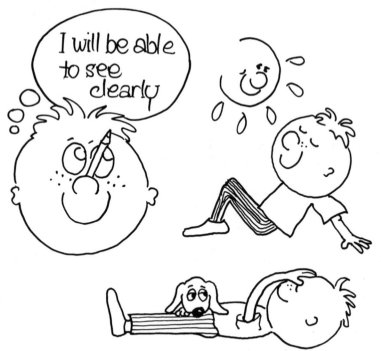

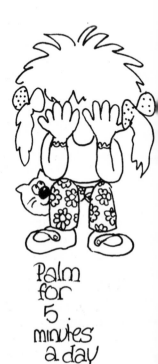

attention from close to far. Create your own mandalas mentally and on paper. See chapter 9.

Support your thoughts. From the discussions on thinking and emotional patterns in chapters 2 and 3, write down your own insights, realizations and affirmations. Adapt this process to your daily life.

CLEARING THE CLOSE BLUR: FOR HYPEROPIA AND PRESBYOPIA

Activate 'edging' and 'sketching' all the time. In addition to your continuous gentle movement, pick up something occasionally. Hold it close for edging. It could be a flower, a pebble, a leaf, your watch, your own or someone else's hand. See chapter 6, p. 49.

Make friends with the near-far swing and use it often. Let it become part of your life. Do it for a few moments interwoven with your reading, sewing, office work, cooking. See p. 52.

(If you are eager to begin using the natural vision methods for clearing your reading, then hop on to chapter 14, Clear Easy Reading Close and Far.)

Palm minimally for five minutes a day to rest your eyes. Visualize images up close as your relaxation increases. See chapter 7, p. 63.

Support your thoughts. From the suggestions in chapters 2 and 3, write down your own insights, realizations, and affirmations. Integrate your own positive thoughts into your daily life patterns.

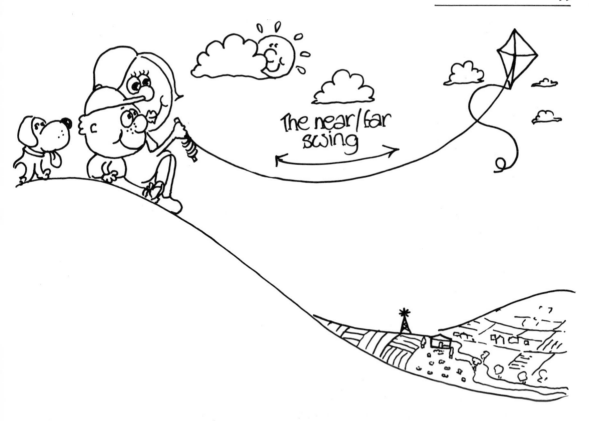

The near/far swing

Blurred vision at all distances can come from increasing dependence on magnifiers and bifocals. It also happens with high degrees of any of the different types of refractive error. This challenging situation means that you get to do all the wonderful vision improvement games mentioned so far. However start yourself off simply. Do the three basics first — edging with nose pencil, sunning and palming. Give yourself plenty of time for change.

THE PAINTING PICTURES GAME: FOR EXPANDING RANGE OF CLARITY

Let us release ourselves from the notion that vision can only be gauged or improved on black and white letter charts. Let's give our sight and ourselves an opportunity to gain confidence in clearing vision by using happy, colorful, pleasant images (photographs of nature for example). Later on we will take this growing confidence in our seeing to the letter charts, then on to motor vehicle or optometric test cards. Do be alert to the sneaky urge to try to see. Transform trying with a big yawn and one of your easy seeing thoughts (such as, 'Everything is coming to me'). If you are using

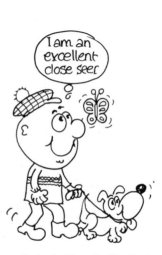

I am an excellent close seer

Seeing for Yourself a First Basic Program

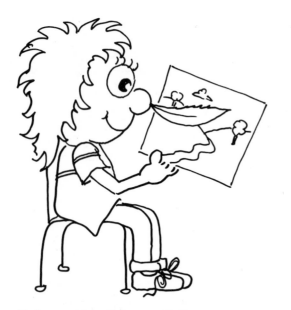

THE PAINTING GAME:
the relaxation and brain
integration that comes
from this simple activity
is one of the best ways
to 'turn on' your eyesight

T-glasses this Painting Pictures activity is good for increasing clarity through those glasses.

Find a photograph or painting that you like. Take a scene from nature. Panoramic vistas of mountains, rivers and spacious skies, flowers or animals are suggested, or use this book's cover.

Sit comfortably and hold the picture you've chosen in your hands. *Put* your nose feather on and scan your image from side to side, from top to bottom, several times. Let your mind be receptive. Absorb the impressions coming to you from the scene. Do this for two or three minutes.

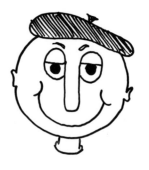

Close your eyes. Put your *magic paint brush* on the end of your nose. It paints with whatever color your mind is talking about at the moment. It gets long or short as need be.

Pretend that your whole visual field is a gigantic canvas. *Paint* in your visual field your current impressions of the landscape and scenery you have just absorbed. Start with the large spaces of color first — the sky, the mountains. Then proceed to smaller details. Feel free to add in any details or hues you would like to put into your landscape. Add animals, flowers or falling snow, galloping horses. You are imaginatively taking off from your experience with the photograph or painting. After you have had a good time painting, *open* your eyes. *Scan* the photo once more. Notice that it may have acquired some new qualities while your eyes were closed, while you were playing with its potentials. The colors may appear brighter. Details may jump out at you. It may be more three-dimensional. It may appear real and alive. The light and shadows may have more contrast. If any or all of these things are true, then you have boosted your visual acuity. The relaxation and brain integration that comes

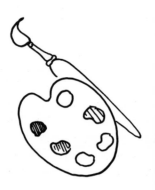

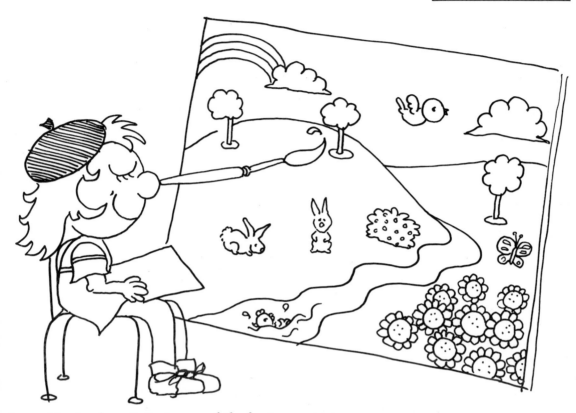

from this simple activity is one of the best ways to turn on your eyesight. It is essential that you 'get into' this game and enjoy the process. If you forget about the time, you know you're into it. Then the usual question of 'How long will it take me to improve my vision?' becomes obsolete. The real question is 'How much vision do I want today?'

The *painting game* can be repeated several times in a row. Each time another layer of detail and clarity will emerge. The flat, two-dimensional photo will come so alive you'll think you have taken a trip to the country.

After you have played this game with photos, transfer the whole process to other things — a tree in your garden, a potted plant in the house — anything that you would like to see light up.

The harvesting of this activity will happen by itself. Completely spontaneous clearing or flashes of vision will happen. It is as if you have given permission to your innate vision to come out and greet the world. Play and enjoy yourself.

LET'S PLAY FAVORITES

I'm imagining that you are in favor of pleasure at this point in your life. I'm seeing you doing those things for yourself that contribute to your happiness, health and inner expansiveness. This allows me to suggest that you choose your favorite activities and do them most often. These will be the activities that you cosy up to most readily, that you fall into easily just because you enjoy the feelings and thoughts that percolate through you when you do them.

Write down your favorites of all the basic activities. When you have made your list, do some sketching of 'This is what I look like when I'm doing my favorite activity'.

_____

_____

_____

_____

DO THE MINIMUM

If you come home from work tired and frazzled, you may feel it's too much work to do these vision activities.

Let me assure you that these relaxing actions are the opposite of work. When you're fatigued, they will rest and energize you.

Sit in a chair and yawn for a while, or lie down and palm. Draw languidly, with eyes closed, the simplest shapes. Do just what you are able to do. Soon you will find the irritation and fatigue of the day dropping away from you. Never mind the eyecharts, the paraphernalia. You will use these at another time when you are more peppy. Now is the time to *relax and rest* with quiet movement and minimal imagery.

Let your mind open up to the idea that less may actually be more. Begin right this moment to make small changes. Add a new habit here and there in your own fashion. These small integrative actions will eventually add up to a new visual beingness.

Chapter 11.

Nuclear Vision

A speck on a ladybird's wing, the moons around Jupiter — human eyes have the potential for seeing these fine details, near or far, thanks to the existence of the fovea centralis, a special area of the retina where the cone cells, our color and detail receptors, are packed closely together to create a point of ultra-sensitivity to light. When the light beams from the object we are looking at fall into the fovea centralis, the visual brain is drenched with millions of bits of data about that object. In fact the visual brain has allocated 35 times more space to the input from the fovea centralis than to any other part of the retina. When the light beams from the object we are mentally attending to scatter or fall somewhere other than into the fovea our vision becomes blurred. The flashes of clear vision experienced by natural vision students occur when their relaxed, responsive nervous system keeps their vibrating eyes and their receptive minds together. If the physical, visual apparatus is represented by the brass section, and the conscious mind by the woodwinds, let's have them playing their music from the same place in the same score.

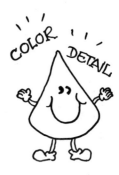

Dr Bates drew our attention to the tremendous acuteness of vision possible when the sight is, as he termed it, 'centralized' or 'centrally fixated'. Because of the tremendous number of cones (from 16 to 20 million) in the fovea each capable of sending its own distinct message into the visual cortex, our vision is able to achieve a level of clarity that could be described as 'ultra' vision. Students describe it in glowing terms. 'The colors and flowers in the garden were resplendent.' 'I'd never seen anything so distinctly before.' 'The sign way across the park jumped out at me.' Words become inadequate. When completely harmonized, vision turns on and it is like being in another state of consciousness. The centring of the vision is a permeating experience — a gentle ecstasy.

I'd like to suggest another term to represent the experience of clear centred vision. Rather than using Bate's phrase 'central fixation' (the eyes are never *fixed* on a point, but vibrate around it) or 'centralizing' let's call the process 'nuclear' vision.

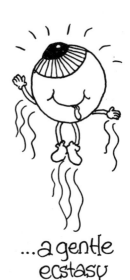

...a gentle ecstasy

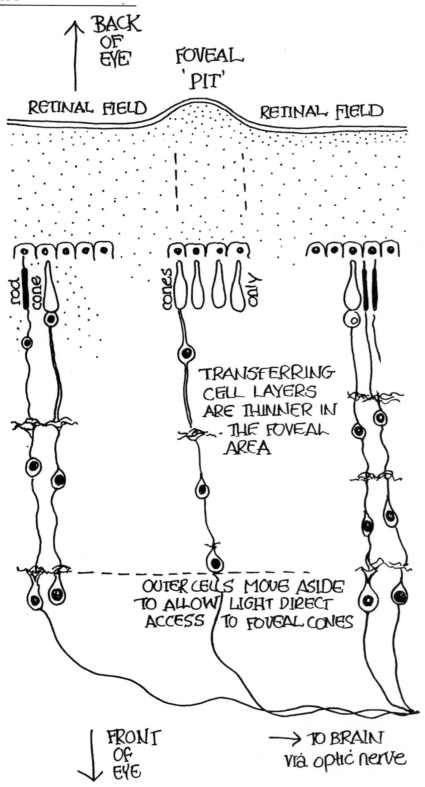

BACK OF EYE

FOVEAL 'PIT'

RETINAL FIELD

RETINAL FIELD

rod cone

cones only

TRANSFERRING
CELL LAYERS
ARE THINNER IN
THE FOVEAL
AREA

OUTER CELLS MOVE ASIDE
TO ALLOW LIGHT DIRECT
ACCESS TO FOVEAL CONES

FRONT OF EYE

TO BRAIN
via optic nerve

Notice that nuclear vision has to do with a oneness in a multitude, a tiny clear center surrounded by a large hazy field. The nucleus of your vision at any moment is the smallest detailed area, the 'apple of your eye', the subject at hand, the most important point of information or appreciation. It reminds me of the 'Hot potato' of childhood games. It is the centre of the energy cyclone that your saccadic movements are constantly perpetuating in your vibrating eyes. This nucleus will feed information to your brain until the mind has all the data it wants or needs from a particular area. Then on to a new nucleus. The speed at which nuclear vision takes place is based on the speed and flexibility of the saccades, (see chapter 6 to review the importance of saccadic movements). The anatomical side of nuclear vision is the large overall area of your retina contrasted to the small region called the macula and within the macula the tinier cone-filled fovea centralis.

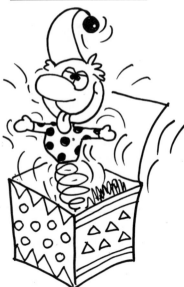

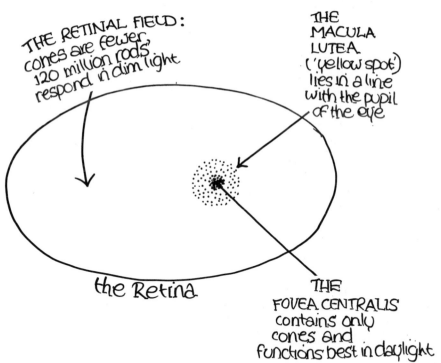

THE RETINAL FIELD:
cones are fewer,
120 million rods
respond in dim light

the Retina

THE MACULA LUTEA ('yellow spot') lies in a line with the pupil of the eye

THE FOVEA CENTRALIS contains only cones and functions best in daylight

In the beginning, play the *nuclear vision* games where you see most easily. (If you have blur everywhere do the game at your natural reading distance.) This is an *emphasis* activity. You consciously affirm what exists — the contrast of field and centre that constitutes nuclear vision. After you have emphasized nuclear vision, it will begin to happen on its own while you're walking down the street, driving the car etc. It could happen anywhere any time in your daily meanderings. What a thrill!

THE NUCLEAR FINGERS

We are able to induce and encourage nuclear vision with simple activities.

Place your pointer fingers approximately 12 inches in front of you and 12 inches apart. Outline your right-hand finger with your nose pencil.

Notice the difference between this finger which is privileged to be receiving both your physical and mental attention at the moment, and the left-hand finger.

The left-hand finger is *less 'nuclear' less vivid, distinct, colorful, alive, detailed, clear.* (If this visual difference between the two fingers is not apparent to you, move your fingers farther apart until a noticeable difference does appear.)

At this moment your right-hand finger is the turned on nucleus of your vision. *Notice* you still perceive all the surroundings — the floor, the walls, the carpet, the ground. They all share the same quality as your left-hand finger. You see them and are aware of them but not in a *nuclear* way.

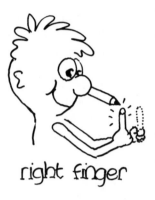

right finger

'Well, this is fine and dandy', one might say. 'Here I am with a nuclear situation but I am getting tired of sitting here only seeing one glowing finger. How do I get *nuclear* vision with something else?'

Easy. You simply move your nose pencil and mental attention to something else. Let's go for the other finger so it doesn't feel left out for too long.

Quickly switch your nose pencil over to the left-hand finger. Notice that this one now lights up and the right-hand finger is turned off, dingy and dull. Switch from finger to finger a few times. Bring the fingers closer and closer together noting the contrast between them. Impress yourself with this simple but significant phenomenon. Delight in your ability to make things distinct and indistinct in your visual field. Chuckle a bit as you play with the electrifying power of your nose pencil. Wherever it goes that place turns on, lights up, becomes the nucleus. Everything else turns off. This process is automatic, inherent to relaxed seeing. The more you encourage it with these short simple activities, the more it will happen by itself.

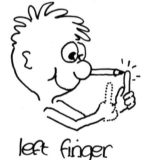

left finger

After you've established your awareness of the nuclear process with two fingers, let's expand it with:

THE GENERAL ELECTRIC GAME

Everything in the universe has a light bulb inside it. Every object, person, cloud in the sky is potentially electric for you, each part of each thing has its own tiny light bulb. All the light bulbs in the universe can turn on for you, brilliantly, one at a time, sequentially,

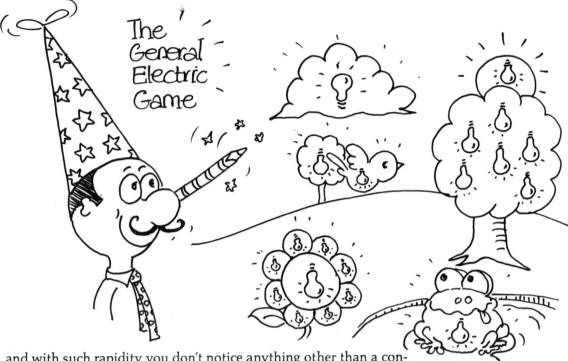

The General Electric Game

and with such rapidity you don't notice anything other than a continuous flow of clear vision.

If you have blur, all the light bulbs are equally turned off. There is no center, no nucleus of clarity anywhere.

How do you turn on the light bulb living inside something? You touch it, encircle it, sketch it with your magic nose pencil which has now graduated to the status of *magician's wand.*

Let's have some magic wand action. Hold up one finger in front of you. Draw the tip of your finger with your nose wand. *Tell* everything else to 'turn off'. Everything else doesn't disappear, it just dims down a little, just like an ordinary light bulb does when it's not plugged in.

Everything, the whole grouping of stuff (shapes and images) around your fingertip, is turned off while your mental attention, your magic pencil wand is turning on the light bulb in the tip of your finger.

Swish your magic pencil wand down to your knee. Now you can truthfully affirm that everything surrounding your knee is turned off (including the aforementioned fingertip). 'Everything else is turned off. '*Turn off,* you stuff!' 'Please turn off, the rest of you shapes.' '*Yes,* indeed, the background, the field surrounding the nucleus that is my knee is turned off'. Repeat these thoughts as you magically switch on the light bulbs in other objects around you.

Continue sashaying about the environment with your magic pencil wand, affirming the turned-off light bulbs, appreciating the brilliant nucleus of your vision. Do this for three or four minutes

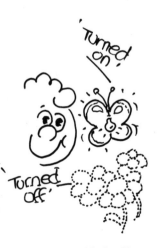

Nuclear Vision

each day (longer if you like). The emphasis and affirmation of nuclear vision will send a message to your visual system, 'Hey, everybody, I've stopped trying to see everything clearly at the same time and the tension is gone'. Your visual system wants to see clearly using its normal and natural capacity for nuclear vision.

We have experienced nuclear vision in relationship to physical eyesight. Use the General Electric game with your eyes closed as well to bring coherency into your inner adventures and movies. Use exactly the same process of telling surrounding images to turn off which permits the one nuclear image to turn on.

What you're interested in accomplishing at the moment will determine your points of nuclear vision. You may wish to locate an opening in traffic or the bananas in a supermarket.

FINDING

To find something you have to recognize it. You can only recognize what you have a mental image of. When you do find the thing you've been imaging and perhaps desiring, the electromagnetic image in your mind connects with the physical object that configuration represents. Let's explore this action further.

If you want to find something, form a picture of it in your mind. Paint it in color and detail, eyes open or closed. Then scan the environment using the handy feather or paint brush. If the object is there it will jump out at you. It's attracted to its similitude in your mind.

If you want to find the scissors in the catch-all drawer, *image* the scissors in the back of your mind and scan the drawer. They will 'pop' out at you. If you want to find your kid in a crowd visualize the color of her/his sweater and scan the area.

HIDDEN PICTURES GAME

Hidden pictures is an example of nuclear vision. Whatever you imagine, your eyes tend to recognize. Accompanying this recognition is a 'flash' of clarity. Playing this game assures your visual system that it's OK to experience things jumping out of the background.

Put the picture 'Mermaid Lagoon' in front of you. Close your eyes and sketch a mermaid. Once her image is recalled and in your mind, open your eyes and scan 'Mermaid Lagoon'. Allow the mermaids to pop out at you.

Follow the same procedure outdoors in nature — with cloud shapes, rock faces, colors on your landscape photos, letters on your eyechart.

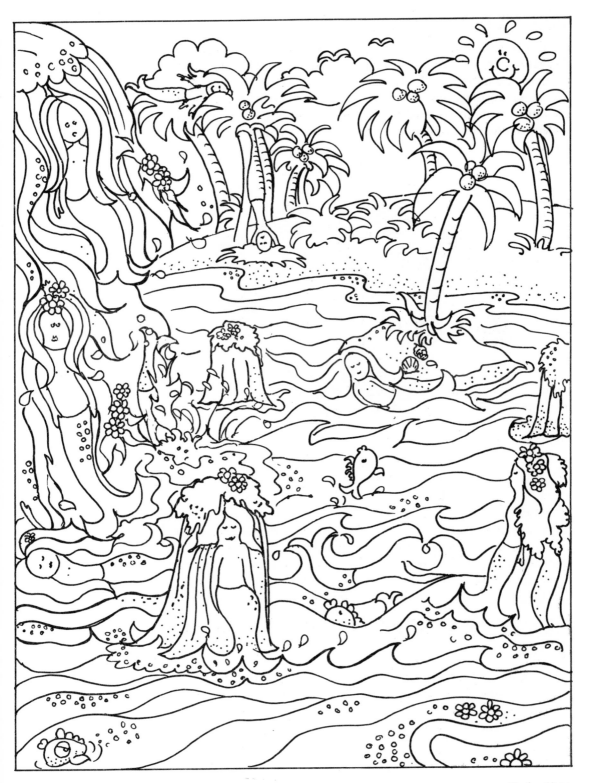

Nuclear Vision

THE COUNTING GAME

Nuclear vision with its ability to single out, if only for a second, a specific item or part of an item is a prerequisite to the ability to count. Counting has to do with discrete *ones* which, when lined up, are willing to receive other names, such as two, three, the second, the third, etc. Emphasizing the process of counting with the visual system can inspire automatic nucleation when you're not thinking about it.

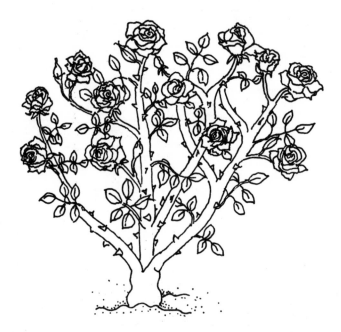

Place the picture of the rosebush in front of you. Sweep across the whole bush then circle each rose in turn with your nose and give it a countable name. One rose, two roses, three roses, etc. in any language you choose. Each rose at the moment of its count assignment will jump forth for you to present its light and glory. Do this process outdoors and eventually with eyechart letters as well.

NUCLEAR VISION IN THE RANGE OF BLUR

I have said up until now that the nuclear games are best played in your clearest vision range. This is done to avoid the tendency to force nuclear vision where it is not happening. However, once you understand the principle and have some experience with the phenomenon of nuclear vision under your belt, experiment with doing it in the blur.

If your blur is in the distance, go out and find some large differentiated shapes. For example, standing in my front yard I see the difference between the soft blue sky, the house across the street and a lofty sycamore tree. I edge the tree and tell the house and sky to turn off their inner lights as in the General Electric games. Then I switch my nose pencil to the house and ask the other two large shapes to turn off. Do this process with colors as well. A large football field swarming with high school bands grouped by their distinctively colored uniforms would be another good opportunity for developing nuclear vision with large blocks of color. A hill, a cloud, a sky are fair game for spacious nuclear vision. Tell the hill and sky to turn off their brilliance allowing the white cloud to entertain your central vision for a time, then trade for the hill or the sky.

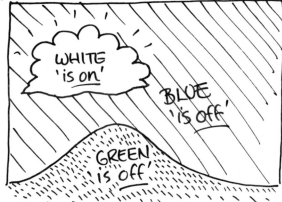

If your blur is up close, you might play the General Electric game with different colored buttons, spools of thread or wool tied around your fingers. Do it with pebbles, leaves, small pictures held in your hand.

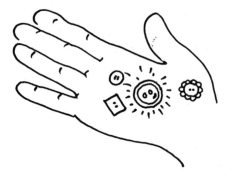

Chapter 12

Seeing with the Whole Brain

I resisted it for a long time. 'Too simplistic', I said. 'Not enough is known. The brain is so complex.' I left the question of left and right hemispheres alone for a long time. It ignored me as well. Then one day someone showed me a brain game that made sense. I was able to literally experience the effects of having both sides of my brain 'switched on'. And the game theory behind the switching on process filled in some gaps for me that had resulted from working with vision students. Here was a missing link to heighten the success of teaching natural vision. My friend, Paul Dennison, was teaching dyslexic children to read and write fluently using an amalgam of muscle testing, meridian balancing and 'cross-crawl' to relink brain circuits. With the whole brain switched on, any learning, re-learning, healing, acquisition of new skills, or unblocking of inherent creativity becomes easier. The stress of trying dissolves away as we experience the innate genius and capacity for growth that blazes through early childhood.

The whole brain theories also answered some questions about incentive. Some students spent several hours a day activating and integrating their vision games in an original way. These students would have clear flashes regularly, pass their driving tests, and be highly enthused. Already 'switched on', they picked up the program and ran away with it, to everyone's satisfaction. Other students would go about it with half a mind, wanting to see clearly yet not activating the program for mental or emotional reasons. Their enthusiasm for the undertaking was being diverted by unconscious homolateral patterns that the gentle optional teaching style of natural vision didn't penetrate. These people were not lazy or stupid as they sometimes announced. They simply wanted 'switching on'.

Could it be that the myopes and hyperopes who had become entrenched in glasses were defending the blur through 'switched off' brain habits? I had thought long about the character aspects of myopia and hyperopia which are discussed in chapter 2 and 3.

Yet character is held in place by the nervous system. Reactive habits, no matter what their origin, are gelled in the current brain/mind patterns. They continue to 'act out' long past the time when the defensive fortifications were first built from necessity. It is far easier to remodel those old bastions when the whole brain is filled with energy, when your analytical voices are in consultation with your universal intuitive voices.

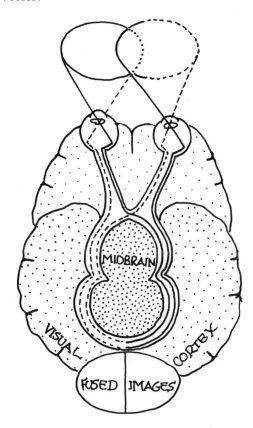

RIGHT-BRAIN AND LEFT-BRAIN

For many years it has been known that the nerve messages from the retinas of your eyes are relayed back to the visual cortex at the back of the head. In more recent studies it has become apparent that other parts of the brain contribute to the process of seeing. Vision is related to intellectual thought, total body coordination, emotions and orientation in space. The home bases for these correlating functions were tracked down through split-brain studies done by neurologists in America. A model emerged that echoed the age-old concepts of polarity and the basic paradoxes of human life. Here is a schematic diagram depicting the division of function between the left and right hemispheres of the human brain. Please remember that these drawings and maps are a simplistic metaphor for the complex interweaving that's actually happening.

Left-Brain Functions	Right-Brain Functions
Right hand control	Left hand control
Hearing	Sight
Awareness of time	Awareness of space
Numbers skills	Music appreciation
Concluding	Initiating
Taking apart	Putting together
Tension	Relaxation
Reasoning and logic	Intuition and psychic perception
Introversion	Extroversion
Convergence	Divergence
The Rational	The Emotional
The Objective	The Subjective
Trying hard	Letting it come
Learning new things	Automatic habits
Attending to specifics	Seeing the whole picture
Written language	Insightful ideas

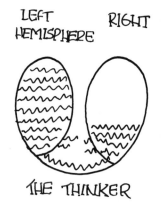

LEFT HEMISPHERE   RIGHT

THE THINKER

SWITCHING OFF AND SWITCHING ON

The top figure is an analogy for someone who is thinking all the time, trying to see, in a myopic state, under body and emotional tension, eats compulsively, has tremendous energy and potential but it is tied up in a knot. (This person could be born right- or left-brain dominant.)

The second figure shows The Dreamer. This is someone who tends to switch to the right hemisphere and spends too much time in a 'spaced out' state. They get overwhelmed in large department stores and have to go home. They make wonderful mystics. To get specific is painful. They tend to be hyperopic, loving to spread their mind into space, dreaming and weaving.

It is possible to swing from one side of the brain to the other, being over-specific and irritable at one time, 'spacy' at another.

The question of dominance of one hemisphere over the other often comes up. We are apparently born with a tendency to be more comfortable with creativity and music than with maths and analysis or vice versa. Those right-brain (dreaming) people in a left-brain (analytical) culture can often trace their unhappiness to being implicitly put down or feeling out of place amongst the 'go get 'em' scientists and business folk. It helps greatly to understand our

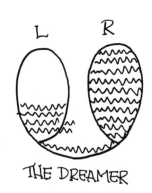

L   R

THE DREAMER

dominance patterns. Yet the most important factor whether you are right hemisphere intuitively inclined or left hemisphere analytically oriented, is *integration* of the two hemispheres in daily life. This makes for a self-realized person, one who is happy, healthy and creative in the total sense. When integrated, we are able to see an image and describe it as well. We want to maximize the flow of energy from one side of the brain to the other and create dual dominance — full activity and interchange of both hemispheres.

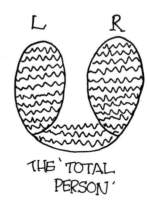

THE 'TOTAL PERSON'

The figure on this page represents someone who is functioning at full capacity. Both hemispheres are 'on', contributing to the overall ability to respond and be responsible in all areas of life with ease and enthusiasm.

In vision classes this person is probably not myopic or hyperopic, but could be dealing with presbyopia or certain stresses in their life. This person probably eats a balanced diet, is healthy beyond the norm, learns quickly and makes comments like 'Yes, I do my vision activities every day. If I say I will do something there is no reason for me not to, is there?' This is the self-starter, an autonomous being who is open to new ideas and carries them through.

The original reasons for switching, going into homolateral patterns, could be physical illness as a child, emotional stress, birth trauma, the effort made to please others, or any of the psychological reactive games we play in order to define, suppress, or survive in our life.

It has been discovered that switching is related to the amount of crawling done as an infant. This period (from 8 to 10 months onward) is when our perception systems are being organized to cross the body's midline. Crawling readies us for the eventual acts of reading and writing where our eyes, hands, and mind will flow from left to right across the midline of the paper.

The act of crawling gave us an explosion of autonomy. We became masters and movers in space. Any inhibition of this crucial creeping where we moved right hand in synchronization with left leg (and vice versa) could contribute to the 'switching off' tendencies.

One could be 'switched on' for body movement, able to play tennis well, able to create winning personal relationships and still be 'switched off' for their eyesight. Someone else could be hassled with food sensitivity, inability to express their personal feelings freely, but integrated for their visual system. The challenge is to recognize our unique switching patterns and to utilize the ways which help to achieve full brain activity. Those of us who became inveterate switchers (jumping into one side of the brain or the other) are able to turn ourselves into 'switcher-onners'. The more we do this the more we learn about ourselves and are able to understand and activate health and happiness in others. Being a 'switcher' is an opportunity to learn and grow.

FIRST MOVE TOWARD SWITCHING ON

The first step to switching on is to return our attention to the nervous system and crawl. Literally get down on the floor and crawl if you like. We also have an integrating movement that can be done standing as well — the cross-crawl. Stand up. Lift your right arm and left leg at the same time. Put them down. Lift your left arm and right leg at the same time. It is that simple. When you physically make this movement you activate both hemispheres of your brain at the same time. You might find this awkward at first. This is the clue that you might be a switcher and did not crawl enough as an infant. Even if you are an athlete, your physical prowess could express itself more easily with less mental effort and fewer accidents or injuries if you begin cross-crawling regularly. Do the cross-crawl to music. If you look up to the left with your eyes and make a counterclockwise circle there, your right brain will be stimulated. If you look up to the right, your left brain will be stimulated. Ultimately we want your gaze to move freely through space in all directions while you are cross-crawling.

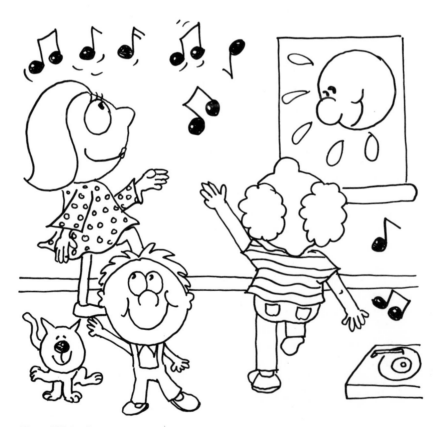

Natural Vision Improvement

Since most people with blurred vision have put effort into their seeing, the general instruction is to cross-crawl looking up to the left for 30 seconds, then generalize the vision by drawing a lazy eight or infinity sign with your nose pencil while cross-crawling. This mental 'crossing' while matching the 'cross' you are making physically with your body switches on mind, eyes and body all together.

Precede your vision improvement games with three minutes of cross-crawling (for maximum effectiveness of those games).

Cross-crawl anytime you feel 'switched' — irritated, uninspired, tense, unable to cope, tired, blocked, blurry, nervous, 'scattered'.

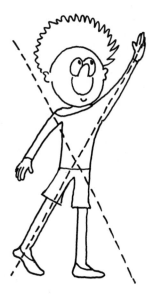

BRAIN VARIATIONS

Some people become so ingrained with the habit of being homolateral, using one side only, that more personal attention is required to sort out and alter their patterns. These people would not be strengthened by the cross-crawl until some other adjustments are made. More information about the availability of practitioners who work in this area can be found. See OTHER RESOURCES page 206. Also, 5 percent of the population are housing their ordinarily right-brain functions on the left side of their head and vice versa (otherwise the world would be monotonous). These people look up to the right to stimulate imagery and spatial rhythm, up to the left to stimulate verbal expression and maths.

Do your best to decide for yourself if you get switched on by glancing up to the left (or edging counterclockwise) or by looking up to you. If you suspect you fall into the overtight, overconcentrated, over-alert area, do your nose movements, edging and sketching generally in a counterclockwise direction. If you feel you are generally balanced, go counterclockwise to enhance your already terrific self.

If you tend to go foggy, mushy, dreamy, then let your movements generally go clockwise. If this doesn't help you to feel more balanced and integrated, experiment with moving into the opposite direction and do your best to find an instructor of Natural Vision Improvement, Touch for Health, or Educational Kinesiology. Check the Appendix for more avenues to practitioners in these areas.

You have moved into an integrated 'switched on' state if any or all of the following things occur:

1. Vision brightens and clears.
2. Breathing loosens and slows.
3. A feeling of harmony comes to you.
4. Your neck and shoulders relax.
5. The world appears more gentle and welcoming.
6. A sense of trust in your ability arises.

SWITCHING ON IN OTHER WAYS

To clear emotional disturbances, hold the frontal eminences. Think about the situation you are gnawing over, run through all aspects of its possible outcome, the fears involved, visualize it to the end. Feel its heaviness lighten as your great 'problem solver' brain says 'All is well and will be happily resolved.' Combine holding frontal eminences with the transformation of images learned in chapter 7. Your fingers act as magnets to draw the brain power forward into both right and left hemispheres from the base of the brain stem where energy may have become lodged in a fear or anxiety reaction.

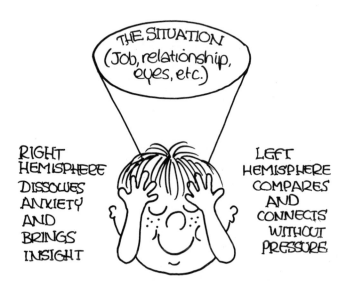

With your fingertips press gently on your brow. Your fingers are calling life energy through your creative brain which has access to intuitive solutions. These inspirations are then flowing across to your left-brain where they can be formulated and expressed in a practical manner. It is the *concern about* the situation that is being dissolved. As the worry lessens your left-brain has a relaxed space in which to clearly analyze the situation and come up with solutions.

Now we get a chance to discover the unconscious resistances that may have dampened your motivation in relationship to improving your vision. Often in classes we ask people to say, 'I want to improve my vision' then discover their body muscles go weak. They are revealing that the thought of seeing clearly is actually switching them off for some hidden emotional reasons. Also, there is a lack of conviction in their voice that exposes an underlying vacillation.

The student holds the frontal eminences for a minute or two while silently running the thought through the mind 'I want to see clearly without glasses', 'I am able to see clearly without glasses', even 'I am able to see clearly *now* without glasses'. The energy reappears in the right hemisphere in company with the thought of clear vision and the person's body muscles become strong when they say out loud 'I want to improve my vision'. The timbre of the voice during the pronouncement becomes noticeably stronger and 'rings true'.

When people are tense or anxious for any reason they may suddenly switch. Certain environments, tasks, or situation may be the trigger points that leave you feeling less than optimum. Be alert to some of the possible factors in your life that can switch you off. For example:

1. Visual Environments, e.g. cheap synthetic carpets in department stores, fluorescent lighting, pictures of life-destructive images, 'negative' environments, even up and down striped wallpaper (a symbol of visual homolaterality).
2. Emotional Exchanges, e.g. people being angry with you, disapproving, doubting, people being impersonal, people who are unloving, officious, stern, people being unresponsive to you.
3. Nutrition, e.g. sugar could do it or wheat, eating when you are tired, eating in social settings.
4. Personal Professional, e.g. when you have to talk about yourself, justify your existence to anyone, defend yourself verbally or otherwise, take an exam which determines your life's course, take an eye test.

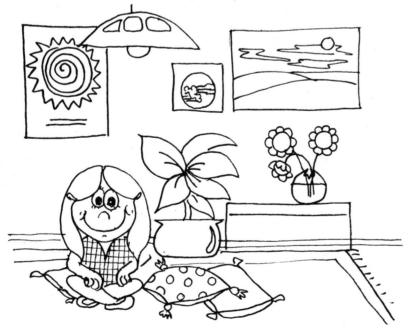

A "switched on" environment

Seeing with the Whole Brain

If you are balanced, integrated and centered in yourself, none of the above will throw you off course, or at least not for long. If you are easily affected, any one of them can cause you to switch to homolateral functioning. To rebalance yourself quickly and effectively I suggest you get involved in the following.

REBALANCING IDEAS

Use body movement: cross-crawling, dancing, walking, running, embracing. Bring in visual symbols: scenes from nature, smiling faces, Xs, flowing patterns, flowers, colors you enjoy. Utilize massage, conscious thought patterns that switch on your whole brain, emotional transformation.

It has been found through muscle testing that the use of certain words and phrases, whether spoken or thought, will affect the current flowing through the hemispheres. For example if you say, 'I can't see', the word 'can't' slams the door on the possibility of something new coming into your life from your unknown abilities, from your right hemisphere.

If you say, 'I am unable to see (so far)', the 'so far' or 'yet' is implied and leaves the door open for changes to happen in the future.

Rather than saying, 'I can't see the sign down the road' or 'I can't read in a dimly lit restaurant', use 'I am unable' and 'able'.

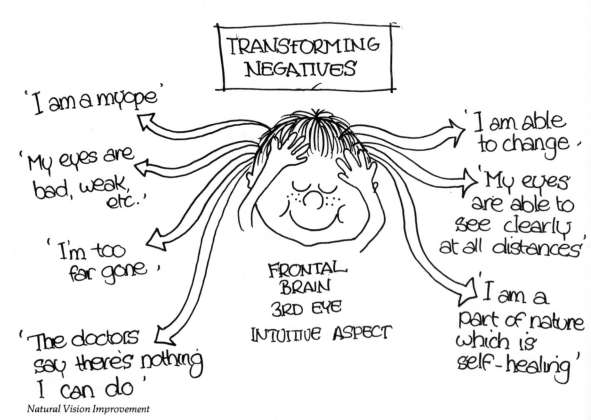

TRANSFORMING NEGATIVES

'I am a myope'

'My eyes are bad, weak, etc.'

'I'm too far gone'

'The doctors say there's nothing I can do'

FRONTAL BRAIN
3RD EYE
INTUITIVE ASPECT

'I am able to change'

'My eyes are able to see clearly at all distances'

'I am a part of nature which is self-healing'

Natural Vision Improvement

Look at these phrases and how they might affect you.

'My eyes are weak.' Don't you feel weak all over with this one?

'My eyes are bad (terrible, poor, etc.)'. Sometimes mothers say this to me within hearing of the child they are describing. 'His left eye is bad.'

'My eyes are beyond hope.' 'There's nothing you can do for me.' (I don't do it anyway, of course.)

Where are these statements coming from? They are all loaded and capable of switching off the ability to change through self-healing.

To strengthen brain integration let's say, 'My eyes are ready for change.' 'My eyes are willing. We are (parent and child) willing to do something about the situation.' 'My eyes will respond. I will respond.' 'Let's go for it, and see what will happen.'

Chapter 13

Fusing Your Eyes
THE FLAVOR OF FUSION

Cover your left eye with your left hand for a few moments. You are now experiencing the visual world as created by your right eye. Move your head around gently, noticing this eye's view of things — the quality, the tones, the feeling. Let's call this world the 'strawberry' world.

Lower your left hand and cover your right eye with your right hand, revealing only the visual ambience conjured by your left eye. It's coming from a slightly different point of view. Colors may be tinted differently and your internal flow of thoughts may have a different nuance. Let's call the left eye view the 'banana' world.

Leave both eyes uncovered. In your mental kitchen let's blend the 'strawberry' and 'banana' worlds together. With your nose sweep through this doubly savory atmosphere. With the energy and messages from both eyes merging together you receive more depth, color, a certain impact not experienced with one eye alone. The whole is more than its parts. Nature has served up this tasteful ability for us to enjoy. The optimum state is for both 'strawberry' and 'banana' worlds to be blended together evenly, simultaneously.

Physically the messages from your two eyes flow through the optic nerves back to the visual cortex at the back of your head. Half of the fibres from each eye cross over at the optic chiasm.

This results in the right visual cortex of the brain receiving data from the left visual field of both eyes. The left visual cortex is sent the messages from the right visual field of both eyes. Our brain then gathers the left visual field input and merges or fuses it with the right visual field. This act of conjoining the two separate data fields is called 'fusion' in this book. This 'first level' of fusion is called 'simultaneous vision' by eye professionals. We will learn more about this in the section on 'The Gate'.

The visual messages continue their journey through the brain to the geniculate body, a midbrain relay point on the way to the visual cortex. The geniculate body sends out notice to other parts of the brain to coordinate eye muscle movements with the data flowing

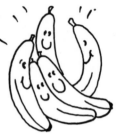

The left-eye view is the 'banana' world

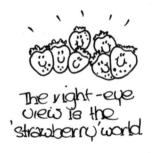

The right-eye view is the 'strawberry' world

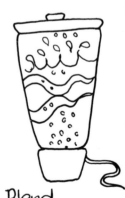

Blend the two together

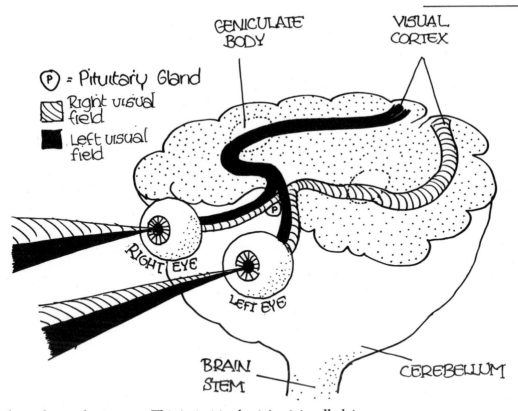

through your brain stem. This 'primitive brain' as it is called, is responsible for organization and communication of all our basic regulatory functions including breathing, pulse rate and alertness. Here also dwell the nuclei that reflexly affect the ciliary muscles of accommodation and eye movements. The midbrain connects as well with the cerebellum (the total brain coordinator and receiver of desires from the conscious mind). The cerebellum assesses the input from the eyes, ears and whole body to create balance and harmony. It also speaks to the autonomic nervous system.

COMING TOGETHERNESS

What is it in the rear of your head that takes separate nerve impulses and creates a stereoscopic image that is vastly different from laying two photographic plates atop one another? What jumps the space between the two sides of your right and left visual cortexes to blend 'strawberry' and 'banana' worlds? No one really knows exactly how fusion occurs. It is complex and wholistic involving many physical and non-physical factors. It is many becoming one-the merging of different elements into a union. It is unmathematical, not just a soup of left eye, right eye impulses mixed together. In my opinion the act of fusion is the contribution of one of our higher vibrational non-physical attributes, namely the creative imagination.

I say this because innumerable times the simple act of students' imagining what they wanted to experience brought about fusion where it had not previously existed, or balanced and strengthened it where it had. We will use this power shortly.

Stress of any sort may have interfered with your remarkable fusing abilities. Let's move step by step to affirm and/or re-establish your fusing abilities.

THE FEELING OF FUSION

Sit comfortably in a chair, with your feet planted on the ground. Or you can sit on the floor cross-legged. Hold your hands in front of you about 2 feet apart, palms facing each other. Take several deep relaxing breaths. Feel the energy radiating from the palms of your hands. Now slowly and deliberately bring your hands together. As they approach each other, interlace your fingers and hold them there. Let your mind receive and absorb the subtle sensations arising from the unity of the hands clasping, the merging of energy. This is what happens in your brain and mind when the disparate messages from your two eyes fuse. Ask for this feeling of union to appear in the back of your head and proceed with the following *Fusion Games*.

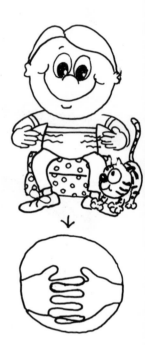

THE GATE — FUSION LEVEL ONE

Put your finger 4 inches directly in front of your nose. With you nose pencil sketch something in the distance.

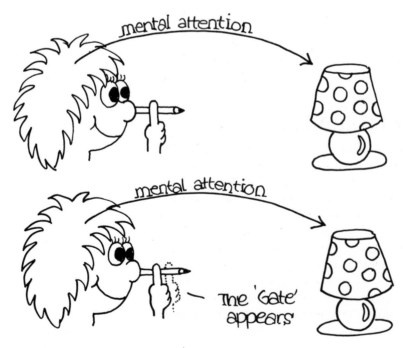

mental attention

mental attention

The 'Gate' appears

While your mental attention is in the distance, you may find that two fingers have appeared. You are now perceiving the 'Gate'. Your brain/mind is fusing the object of attention in the distance and not fusing the finger in front of you. This finger 'gate' allows you to notice the image that enters each eye quite separately. The finger to the right of your nose is the 'banana' world (left eye's) view. The image of the finger to the left of your nose is the 'strawberry' (right eye) world. Because of the cross-over of the fibres at the optic chiasm the object you are paying attention to and edging in the distance is fused, single and nuclear.

I'd like you to notice also that when you bring your attention to your finger that the gate disappears. Instantly and automatically the two fingers merge into one. You have fused the finger. Objects in the distance are now doubled and hazy. Wherever your conscious mental attention goes, fusion takes place at that point in the midst of your fabulous saccadic dancing. Remarkable! When fusion is happening naturally, your visual perception system is functioning without fatigue, aches or annoyance. Efficiency is high and learning easier while your eyes remain relaxed and coordinated.

The appearance of the two fingers is what we want when your attention is in the distance. It means that you have conscious access to the messages from both your eyes. If you have two equal fingers, skip on to the Bead Game. Please be sure that the light falling on your finger is coming in equally from both sides. Otherwise your Gate images may appear unequal when they're actually not.

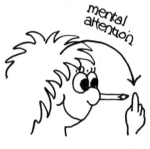

'...the gate disappears'

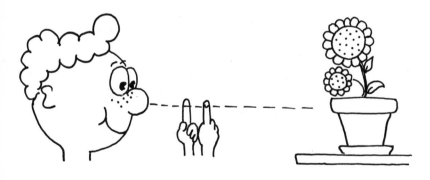

'My fingers are identical twins, I'll go to the 'bead game!'

THE HALO

If you want to strengthen and integrate your unconscious automatic habit of fusion level one in conjunction with developing acuity, make yourself a halo. It replaces the finger, giving your arm a rest.

In America I obtained aluminium plastic-covered clothesline wire which is bendable yet still holds its shape enough to make a halo. (see next page.) Find a similar material if possible, or use a cap with an attached stick. Decorate the cap if you like. Colored plastic tape on the nose piece may interest children who are using their own halos. The halo is excellent for wearing while doing the Bird Dance in chapter 6 (see page 54) as it combines fusion with saccadic movement. It is also good to use for the reading activities in chapter 14.

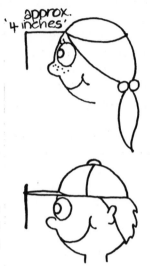

The 'Halo'

approx.
4 inches

WHEN THE GATE IS UNEQUAL

If you have one 'solid' finger and one that appears hazy or 'ghostly' this is an indication of an imbalance in the energy flow through your visual system. Usually the ghostly finger will correspond to an eye that is more tense and blurred than the other. The blurred eye is not 'weaker' or 'bad'. It will respond to relaxation and 'switching on'. To determine which eye to cover, realize that the right image of the Gate belongs to the left eye and vice versa. Patch the eye that corresponds to the strongest side of the Gate. Do some games wearing your patch as on page 134. After unpatching do the following activity.

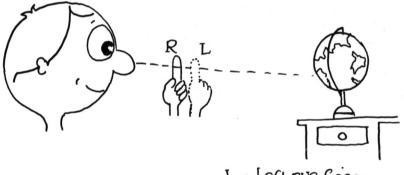

L = Left eye finger
R = Right eye finger

'I have one strong finger and one a ghost. I'll do some patching games'

Palm your eyes and take a trip to a Greek island where ancient ruins dream on high green bluffs against a sky of hot blue. Stand 10 feet in front of two weathered white columns. Visualize the solidity of the marble pillars, one on your left, and one on your right. Sketch the columns with your nose pencil, one at a time. Then imagine the two columns simultaneously while your nose pencil sketches olive trees in the distance between them. The columns are mates, counterbalancing each other, framing the classic scenery between them. Open your eyes and proceed.

Use a brightly colored pen or pencil to make the Gate. Close your eyes and *pretend* that both your pencils, the 'gate posts', are of equal strength. Use your nose paint brush to spruce up the color on each gate post. Keep on painting and visualizing until your mind

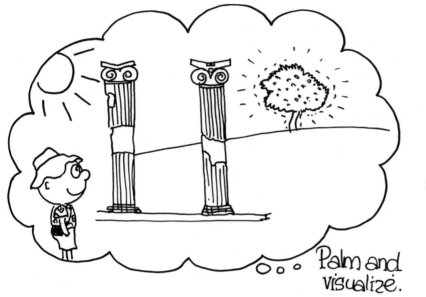

Palm and visualize.

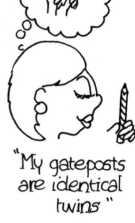

"My gateposts are identical twins"

is persuaded that the two gate posts are identical. Mutter under your breath, 'My gate posts are identical twins.' Maintaining this thought, let your eyes *open*. Go on imagining. You may notice that the images forming the *Gate* are more equal in intensity. Do this activity often until your Gate is balanced.

WHEN THERE'S NO GATE

If you do not have two pencils, i.e. the Gate, it may be that one side or the other of your brain is switched off or 'asleep' (as in amblyopia or squint) and is asking for stimulation. In this case, go to the Patching section of this chapter after doing cross-crawl games from chapter 12. Then return to this page.

It is possible that the Gate may be coaxed into appearing by imagining. Close your eyes and visualize two pencils in front of you. Keep on remembering the appearance of the 'Gate', and open your eyes. Momentarily the two pencils may have appeared together. Do this several times. Always with nonchalance. Sometimes a penlight or candle in a darkened room will give you even more help in calling in the second image of the Gate.

Still no Gate? Then let's make ourselves a 'Fantasic Fusion Fixer'.

Obtain a piece of stiff cardboard about 4 inches wide and 8 inches long. Ideally one side of the cardboard is red and the other side green, or one side is blue and the other side orange, or yellow and violet — always complementary colors. Pasting together two pieces of different colored construction paper might do. Or paint your cardboard. At a pinch, just use plain white paper and proceed to the next step.

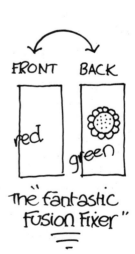

FRONT   BACK

red   green

The "fantastic Fusion Fixer"

Fusing Your Eyes

Glue to one side of the card a picture of a bright flower or animal — anything you wish as long as it contrasts with the background color on that side of the card. Leave the other side blank.

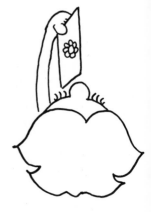

Hold the card in front of your nose snug enough to your face so that your right eye sees only the right side of the card and your left eye sees only the left side of the card. Put the bird or flower next to the eye that wants awakening.

Cover your right eye with your hand. Experience, absorb and memorize the side of the card that you see with this eye.

Cover your left eye with your hand. Experience, absorb and memorize the side of the card you see with this eye.

Now with both eyes closed visualize the left eye's side of the card to the right of your nose. Visualize the right eye's side of the card to the left of your nose. Now imagine the two sides at the same time. I agree it's tricky.

Open both eyes, say 'hurrah' if both sides of the card appeared at the same time, even for a split second. Repeat this activity until you have a solid, lasting experience of simultaneous vision.

WANDERING EYES

Wandering eyes that float either in or out most often result from chronic tension in the large external muscles of the eye. Spasming muscles exert a constant tug in one direction or another preventing the eyes from coordinating themselves.

We might speculate that the nerves innervating the tense muscles would benefit from the freer brain/body communication derived from the cross-crawl and other 'switching on' techniques from chapter 12. Sometimes surgery is performed on wandering eyes and the muscles are clipped. The effect is generally only cosmetic, often unsuccessful. Usually there is no assurance that the surgical invasion will help restore the sight even when eyeglasses and/or orthoptic exercises are used later. If there has been surgery, it might be helpful to take the person (child or adult) back through the unconscious memory of the operation (see page 120) to heal that experience.

All the relaxation games in this book will help to release tight eye muscles including those involved in esophoria (crossed eyes) and exophoria (eyes that swing outward). There are a few people who alternately turn one eye then the other. This kind of situation may require the aid of a certified teacher. However, if a teacher is not available to you, relax yourself with all the general vision activities. Then use every game described in the preceding section 'When There's No Gate'.

All these straying eyes can be helped even further by some specific directional games. Our desire is to end up with both eyes able to vibrate around the same point at the same time.

TROMBONING FOR WANDERING EYES

Make yourself a paddle of stiff cardboard. Because the eyes are always attracted to motion and color we will move the paddle like a trombone to coax the wandering eye in the direction we want it to go. We want the overtight muscles to relax and the supporting nerve supply to flow freely. Put some brightly colored stickers or cutouts on the paddle to attract the eye. (Obtain stickers in children's stores and stationers).

For an eye that tends to drift outward, cover the other eye and hold the paddle in front of you. Trombone the paddle in and out crossing the midline of your body, noticing the picture getting larger and smaller. Hum with the in and out rhythm of the paddle. The humming or crooning sound will vibrate bones and activate the right hemisphere. The paddle attracts and coaxes the eye inward. You might do it with music.

For an eye that tends to pull too far inward, the moving paddle is used to escort the eye in an outward direction. Covering the opposite eye with the palm of the hand, trombone the paddle from the nose outward, away from the midline of your body. Again, humming and crooning will help to stimulate the visual system while easing the eye outward.

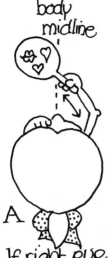
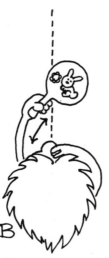
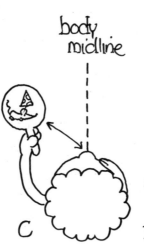
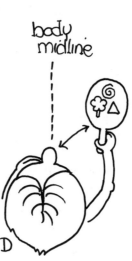

A
If right eye goes out, the paddle moves across your body's midline and outwards to the left

B
If left eye goes out, the paddle moves across your body's midline and outwards to the right

C
If left eye goes in, the paddle moves away from your body's midline to the left

D
If right eye goes in, the paddle moves away from your body's midline toward the right

Fusing Your Eyes

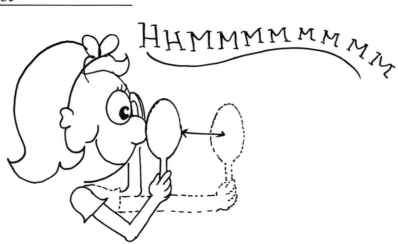

The Paddle travels from arms length to the tip of your nose

If you have at least fusion level one — the Gate — you will be able to enjoy and advance your eye/mind coordination and fusion flexibility with:

THE BUG ON THE BEAD — FUSION LEVEL TWO

Take a piece of string about 5 feet long. Tape or tie one end of the string to a window or chair at eye level. Sit comfortably about 4 feet away and hold the other end of the string in your hand. Keep the string about 6 inches out from your chin so that you can easily move your nose and head. Place a brightly colored bead on your string (or paper clip, ring, piece of yarn, etc). Put the bead 12 inches from your hand.

Now that you are all set with your string and bead, close your eyes and pretend you have a pet bug flying about the room. It could be a butterfly, ladybird, housefly or a more exotic type. Give the bug a color and a name. Imagine the color, size and sound of your bug. This bug is going to keep you loose while you develop precise flexible fusion. Follow it with your nose. It leads your nose a merry chase around the room. It swoops and glides and performs loop-de-loops with the greatest of ease. This bug is a show-off. When it

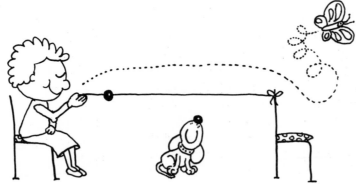

is ready to rest it will gracefully alight on your bead. Draw a small anticlockwise circle on the bug on the bead with your nose. Open your eyes, still visualizing the bug on the bead. Do you notice that when your attention is on the bug and bead that there is a doubling of your string? Two strings are now meeting to make a cross somewhere in the vicinity of your bug and bead. Aha! your gate has turned into a giant X. You're using the messages from both eyes simultaneously and your mind and eyes are together.

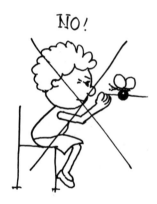

If your X crosses at the bead or close to it, proceed on from here to Flexing with Fusion. If your X crosses considerably beyond or in front of the bead, skip on to the 'Widening River' or 'The Precious Shell' whichever fits your situation.

If at any point in the Bug and Bead game you find yourself stiffening, trying hard or staring, simply take a deep breath, yawn and follow your bug around the room again.

FLEXING WITH FUSION

Trace its aerial adventures and move your bead to another point on the string while bug is in flight. Then bring your bug down again on to the bead. The bug sits and preens itself for a moment. Then it takes off again while you sneak the bead into another position. Do this game several times until you are satisfied with your ability to get an X quickly and easily no matter where the bug lands.

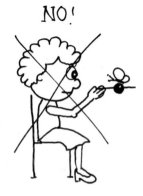

It's time now to let your bug rest on the bead while you do all the movement. Grasp the bead with two fingers and slide it near and far on the string. Your smiling bug holds your attention as it gets a ride. You will see the X zooming near and far, travelling right along with the bead. This action is going to flex your accommodative muscle, changing the shape of your lens for distance and close vision while you are maintaining fusion. If you feel your eyes tightening up as the bead comes in close, use your relaxation abilities to ease away the strain. When you've accomplished facile, agile, free movement with this activity, you need only do it on occasion hereafter.

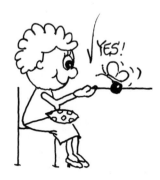

THE WIDENING RIVER

If your string is crossing in front of your bead, your eyes want relaxation outward. They are overconverging. Stop, put down your string, palm, and visualize. Imagine you are standing at the wellspring of a river which widens as it flows away from you. Trace the side of the river extending out to the right and then the side extending to the left. See the figure on the next page.

Take down your hands and pick up your string. With the sensation and image of the widening river in the back of your head, return to the bead. Maybe your X is now on the bead or closer to it.

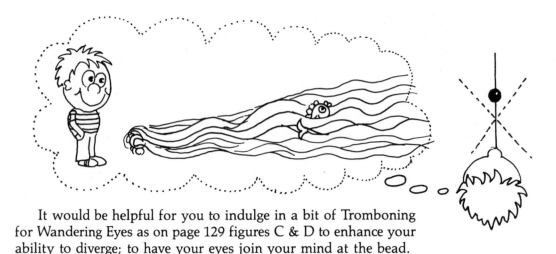

It would be helpful for you to indulge in a bit of Tromboning for Wandering Eyes as on page 129 figures C & D to enhance your ability to diverge; to have your eyes join your mind at the bead.

THE PRECIOUS SHELL

If your string is crossing beyond your bead, your eyes want relaxation inward. They are diverging too much. Stop, put down the string, palm, and visualize. Imagine you are standing on the seashore. Hold a tiny intricate seashell in the palm of your hand. Bring it close to you and examine its beauty for a while. Then open your eyes and continue with the Bead Game.

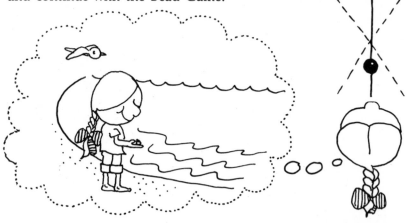

Your X may have fallen closer to your bead. Happy day! The Tromboning for Wandering Eyes on page 129 figures A & B will aid in bringing your eyes inward to meet your mind on the bead.

TAKING FUSION INTO DISTANCE

Sometimes people with blur in the distance will short-circuit their distance fusion as well. It is possible to have balanced fusion up close, but have it waver in the distance. For these people it is a good idea to tape the end of your string to a window. Put your

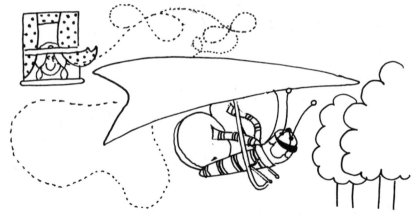

bug on a hang-glider for this one. The bug (dressed in her/his team colors) makes a running slide down the string and sails off into the distance out the window. Now follow happily with your nose like a faithful puppy. Out your hero flies, swooping and doing figure eights into the distance until the exhilarated bug lands on a distant branch where you contentedly circle it with your nose, a tiny circle that you make while affirming the feeling that your eyes are perfectly balanced and fused at that distance. Do this as often as you like to feel completely relaxed and 'together' in the distance.

When doing Bug and Bead, sit relaxed and erect. Relaxed, not collapsed. Yawn a great deal and smile a little.

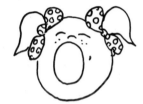

EXPLORATIONS WITH THE PIRATE PATCH

Sometimes we have decided to visually accommodate to the world by creating variations in our eyes. One eye may see clearly in the distance and the other eye clearly up close. Sometimes this discrepancy results in amblyopia where the brain receiving the input from the eye is 'switched off' even though the physical eye is perfectly healthy. Sometimes the retinal messages are still used and people use one eye then the other. The chaos that these imbalances perpetrate in our nervous system is usually suppressed and adapted to, yet it is entirely possible and far better to reactivate the brain with 'Switching on' and give the eyes an opportunity to fuse. See chapter 12 for cross-crawl then let us do Patching with relaxing vision games to 'wake up' the brain. After we will travel back to page 124 to achieve the 'Gate'.

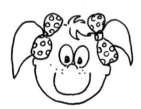

For anyone who wants to hone their vision in each eye separately, playing Pirate with the Patch is an excellent idea. Eye patches can be found in drug stores. If any time patching causes stress then it is counter-productive. Wear the patch for only short periods of time and generally while playing particular vision relaxation games.

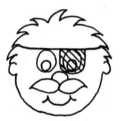

Fusing Your Eyes

SAMPLE ACTIVITIES WITH PATCH

Put on your patch and spend:
5 minutes sunning. Yes, with both eyes closed.
5 minutes edging with the Magic Pencil. Open your eyes and spend:
5 minutes doing a near-far swing
5 minutes Free as a Bird swings
5 minutes Palming, patch off, with images of symmetry and balance.

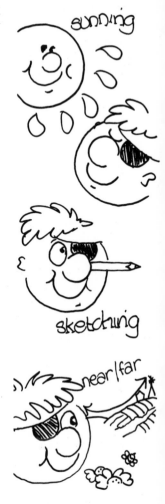

When you patch you may experience the different personalities of each eye and of yourself. Explore the world you create and perceive with each eye separately.

Spend some unmeasured time with a patch on roaming about the yard, sniffing and examining flowers and levels. Sweep, scan, explore the shapes and colors of your territory. It may be a new area in which you'll find some hidden treasure!

Yawn, Yawn, Yawn

When one eye appears to have more challenge with the physical world than the other, give it some of your attention. Talk with it and find out what subtle resistances it may be clinging to. Paint and draw with the patch on. Which eye do you function from most of the time? People sometimes ask me about covering the dominant eye as in right and left hand dominance. There is a dominant eye. It's the one you use for sighting through a telescope or camera lens. It may or may not be the clearer eye. The question of dominance diminshes as we grant ultimate importance to fusion and integration.

Take off the patch. You may switch it to the other eye to play with the clearer eye if you like. After removing the patch, with eyes open or closed, experience the 'Gate' for a few seconds to reaffirm the togetherness of your eyes.

MERGING CIRCLES — FUSION LEVEL THREE

If you have the Gate, it means that your eyes are functioning simultaneously. If your X crosses at the bead (where the mental attention is pausing), then your eye/mind coordination is good. Beyond this are further refinements to fusion which include the ability to bring two slightly disparate images into one by playing with the merging circles. Remember that when the eye muscles point the eyes in the direction needed to pick up corresponding data, it is still the mind that welds the incoming images into a coherent whole. The influence of the mind's attitude is well displayed by playing with the first pair of circles.

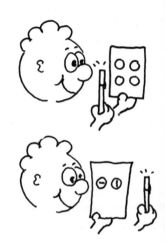

Hold the fourth colour plate about 30cm in front of you. Let your mental point of attention go either beyond or in front of the surface of the page. (Holding your finger or pen to attract your mental attention 6 inches in front or behind the page may facilitate the effect.)

Soon you'll see three circles, the centre one an amalgam of orange and blue. When you murmur the word 'blue' you'll see more of the blue wave length that is bouncing off the paper. When you whisper 'orange', you'll perceive more of the orange color. Color is all in your mind. It doesn't exist outside of your creating and perceiving it, as a simultaneous act.

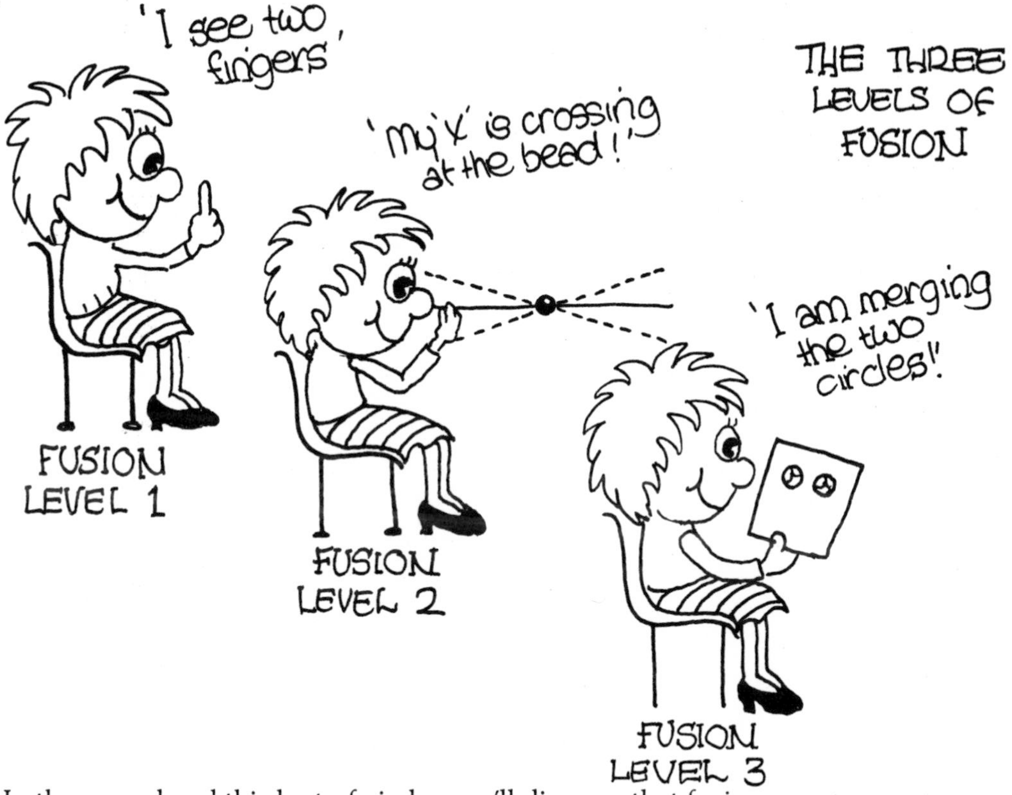

'I see two fingers'

'my x is crossing at the bead!'

'I am merging the two circles!'

THE THREE LEVELS OF FUSION

FUSION LEVEL 1

FUSION LEVEL 2

FUSION LEVEL 3

In the second and third set of circles you'll discover that fusing them together in the manner described above results in a three-dimensional effect. These two slightly different circles are coming in to this wonderful illusion of depth due to your brain's integrating capacity.

Many of us are being led down the technological path to a chair that fronts a computer terminal. The compensation may be monetary for forcing the human eyes and brain to receive the output of electronic data banks. The price is often a disruptive challenge to our stamina and ultimately to our mental and physical health. An Australian optometrist commented 'Nothing could have been more poorly designed for the interface between people and machines than the computer screens in current use.' One specific result of sitting for hours at close range to readout screens and piles of computer print is the depletion of fusional reserve. This is the capacity to fuse easily under all circumstances. Some people have lots of it and are able to function (visually) with relative happiness at a new clerical job. Others don't have as much fusional reserve and end up miserable in their job. Bank tellers, for example, who never had eye disturbances before, find their eyes growing tired, sore, and blurred when their old sheafs of mobile notepads are replaced by a stationary computer screen. If you find yourself in such a dilemma, use the basic relaxation activities in this book at regular intervals throughout the day and play with the Rosebush Path of Circles. (Color plate 4)

Start at the top, fuse those two rosebushes just as you did with the previous circles. Then proceed downward, fusing each pair of rosebushes in turn. By the time you've reached the bottom pair, you will have significantly strengthened your converging fusion ability, a crucial item for lots of close work!

Chapter 14

Clear Easy Reading Close and Far

THE AGONY VERSUS THE ECSTASY

Most of us learned to read between the ages of four and eight. Some of us were ready and eager at age six or seven to sit still for the left-brain concentration necessary for acquiring the new skills of interpreting symbolic language. Some of us were not.

Paul Dennison who earned his doctorate in education speaks about traditional educational procedures, 'Americans seem to have an undying faith in materials and software to solve the literacy problem. Millions of taxpayers' dollars have been spent on innovative reading systems, machines, and computer technology, while ignoring the human machine for which these were all intended. American educators tend to *try to change the child to fit the materials*, compounding the problem, instead of understanding how people can learn better and more successfully.'

If the shoe fits, we could put it on in other countries as well. Those of us who embarked bright-eyed and glossy the first day of school ran into some perhaps still unresolved emotional sandbars where we left our innocent aspirations derelict and unfulfilled. Now when I reach the reading stage in vision workshops and classes, I ask adults to stand up and *read aloud*. The residue of early school experience flares up in reluctance, awkwardness and sudden blurring of the print. Everyone is instantly transported back to the pigtail and woollen sock days. Memories are being regurgitated of certain sour experiences, humiliations, and teasing by teachers and classmates.

One of my most delightful, responsive, and in the beginning, highly myopic students, aged thirty-seven moaned, 'My parents actually thought I was retarded until I was twelve years old. Then I learned to play the piano. For the first time I felt happy about myself. After that I taught myself to read.' An optimistic, spirited woman, aged fifty six, who managed a private school for twenty

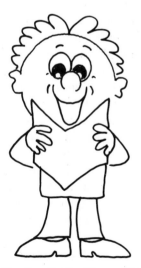

Clear Easy Reading Close and Far

years said, 'All my family members were early readers, except me. No one realized that my older sister read dramatically to me every night before bed. It never crossed my mind that I should learn to read also. So I was the black spot on the family record when I started school.'

We help to resolve those old scars by holding foreheads and saying 'I am a wonderful reader' and 'I am a smashing, entertaining, glorious reader' and 'I love to read and I love to read aloud to myself and to my friends' This is followed by cross-crawl as on page 116 for a couple of minutes.

The alteration in attitude and performance is striking and noticeable to everyone. Adults who have been wearing various types of spectacles for reading are seeing clearly without their glasses, and having a high time reading stories aloud. Often, their long-suppressed joy in reading, drama, and sharing images emerges. Their eyes and minds light up and the print is clear.

Reading is potentially a great joy. It can lead us into halls of learning, arenas of self-expression, and toward superb action in school and business. For unhampered accomplished reading our eyes want to be mobile, fusing well, and easily accommodating (coming to near points with clarity). A fully 'switched on' brain and positive attitude are the first ingredients for revising our reading experience. To this we'll add the 'Great White Glow' — a reading style that harmonizes with visual physiology to keep you out of lenses for the printed word.

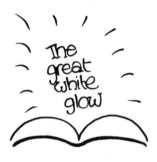

OLD AGE SIGHT, DO WE NEED IT?

The prevailing message is, 'Forty-five years old now? Hmmmm? Arms getting too short? Ha, ha, well we've all seen better days. Time for you to own a nice stylish pair of reading glasses.' It is all part of the natural aging process. The lens of the eye stiffens with age. The only remedy — glasses. Most people succumb. The suggestibility factor is operative. One student whose optometrist friend had told him he'd need reading glasses by the time he was forty-two years old was beset by reading blur on the morning of his forty-second birthday. Ignorance about options prevails. We're not given a booklet on 'How to Retain Accommodative Flexibility' in the opticians' place of commerce. A lot of people fend off the glasses stubbornly, ending up with corrugated foreheads from squinting or unnecessarily sacrificing their love of reading. This is the story except for natural vision students and those who don't believe in aging as culturally programmed. Yes, it is true that there are body changes as we add numbers to our years. Yet many people retain their flexibility of body and mind through exercise and diet. You always have a choice. You either slide with the downhill trend, let muscles go flaccid, accept less than vibrant health and become more sedentary or you can get better as you grow older. You could become even more active, an avid learner, wiser, filled with self-respect. You could become more expressive, utilizing your experiences, becoming healthier as you refine your relationship to life.

It is possible to keep your eyes out of reading glasses just as you can keep your bones out of crutches. The factors to consider when retaining or recovering your reading vision are:

1. *The continued flexibility of your lens*: The lens changes its shape to accommodate, to cooperate with your mind in creating clear distance and clear close vision. When your attention comes close, the lens steepens its curvature. When your attention goes far, the lens flattens. Please consider the fact that your lens never sits still in one place. In a healthy alive state, it is continually pulsating and fluctuating. It does this through its connection to the ciliary muscle which is directed by the hypothalamus, the emotional center of your brain.

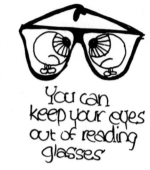

You can keep your eyes out of reading glasses

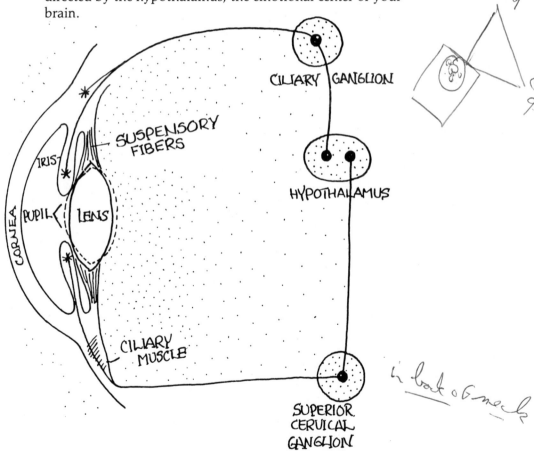

2. *The use of reading glasses*: The use of reading glasses (magnifying lenses) prevents the ciliary muscle and lens from doing their jobs of flexing and relaxing to alter the curvature

of the lens. The reading glasses make the print bigger, preempting the necessity of the lens changing its curvature. When your eyes are behind glasses, you are no longer using your accommodative skills. This is why the adoption of reading glasses is always a trap. Once you begin using them, the muscles and lens become more and more sluggish and less and less able to perform for you. Hence, you are prescribed stronger lenses on your next visit to the eye doctor. Even people who have enjoyed superb visual acuity all their lives begin to lose their distance vision after spending time in magnifying lenses.

NEAR-FAR ON THE PERUVIAN PLAINS

The maintenance and restoration of the flexibility of your lens and accommodation muscles are within your capabilities. This can be done with Near-Far Swings and Tromboning.

You were introduced to some of the benefits of the Near-Far Swing in chapter 6 where we use it in driving and for flexibility of seeing range. Now you can utilize a form of the Near-Far Swing to specifically tone and flex your accommodation skills. Sitting in a chair, close your eyes and imagine:

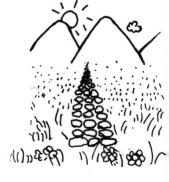

You are resting on the side of a green hill in the mountains of Peru. When you breathe in you inhale the high mountain air. Crystalline pure air. Paint the lucid blue sky overhead with your largest paint brush. The grass spreads around you sprinkled with tiny yellow wildflowers. Sweep through the grass with your paint brush. Feel the tickling effect of those gleaming flowers. The blades of grass tickle your mind. Your eyes are being released to vibrate. Feel the warm sun on your shoulders. Imagine the plains high in front of you spreading into the distance. On these plains are ancient formations made of large weatherworn stones. Trace the edges of these rocks with your nose. The land is flat, giving you an interesting perspective to sketch in with your paint brush. These huge rocks were placed together without mortar. You trace low-lying walls and roadways. In the distance, far across the plains, lie mountains. Trace the violet mountain peaks. Inhale this expansive distance into your mind. Straight in front of you, extending across the plains, you notice a row of flat rocks illuminated by the sun. These rocks form a straight line into the distance. Trace the rocks outward with your nose. When your nose arrives at the farthest point, draw a counterclockwise circle. Now exhale all the air from your lungs, inhale fully and let your nose and attention slide back in on the rocky roadway until your chin comes to your chest. Make a circle on the center of your tummy with your nose. Again exhale and inhale fully. Slide outward again as before into the distance. Move slowly and thoroughly. Distance is inside your head. You can imagine distance and you can imagine close. Grow accustomed to enjoying and activating this near-far action. Your eyes will be delighted.

TROMBONE EXPRESS

Make yourself a paddle. You can purchase one disguised as a ball game for kids in the toy store. Remove the ball and rubber band. Spray paint it all one color. You could also make one using a piece of cardboard. It is helpful if the paddle is a dark color, black or blue, so that the background of the paddle contrasts with the bright colored images that you paste on it.

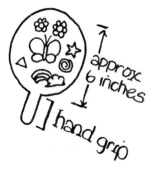

approx 6 inches

hand grip

Decorate your paddle with paper reinforcements, colored dots from stationers and colored stickers (if you're a grandparent, ask your grandchildren to share their sticker collection). Cut-outs from magazines or a phrase or two in print (leave on the white background) are fine also. Be creative with this small project.

Your paddle is meant to be carried with you in your pocket or purse. You could make a few in different sizes because tromboning loves to be done at odd moments.

Palm your left eye with your left hand. Grasp your paddle in your right hand and bring it in and out, near and far, from your nose to the length of your arm. Start this sliding action slowly, then speed up (it will tone your biceps and triceps as well as your ciliary muscles). It is excellent to hum or howl a nonsensical but rhythmical sound in harmony with your in and out motion. You might be surprised at how entertaining this can become, especially if there are some children in the house. Do this action for two or three minutes moving the paddle straight away from your nose or slightly inward. If you have an eye or eyes that wander, refer yourself to Tromboning for Wandering Eyes in chapter 13 page 129.

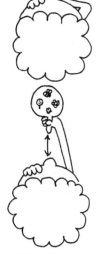

The paddle taps your nose and...

tap!

extends out to arms length on it's in and out motion

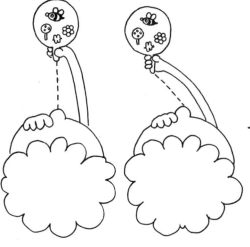

Trombone straight out from the nose or slightly inward

The Tromboning is then switched to the opposite side. Palm your right eye with your right hand and flex the paddle in and out for your left eye.

The tromboning is done for short periods of time, as often as possible. It is a good warm-up for any reading venture. Use it for a few seconds before the morning paper or evening pleasure reading. Use it tune up the accommodative powers before practicing the Thrill of The Great White Glow, your new style of reading that's coming up next.

The benefits of Tromboning are not reserved just for people with reading glasses and 'old age sight'. The Tromboning is useful for short-sighted, long-sighted and astigmatic people. For short-sighted people, the Tromboning activity activates retinal nerves, wakes up visual brain cells and energizes the visual system. For long sighted and astigmatic people, it creates flexibility for seeing clearly at close range.

THE THRILL OF THE GREAT WHITE GLOW

White paper reflects practically all the light that comes to it into your eyes, while black ink absorbs nearly all the light. Because our visual system is activated by receiving light, we see and recognize the shapes of black print by perceiving the white spaces around the letters.

Reading is a situation where we have to revise old assumptions. We were told to 'look at the letter' and 'look at the word' in school. This appeared to assist us in learning to read, as long as the act of looking at the unseeable black print did not interfere with the process of perceiving and utilizing the white space around the letters (even if this aspect of reading was unacknowledged). When we want to restore or relax our reading vision, we give up our straining efforts to see the black and begin to connect strongly with the white surrounding it.

The same concept holds true for eyecharts in the distance. Struggling to see the unseeable black letters results in more tension and blurring. The answer to visual blur on paper at any distance is to become closely acquainted with the virtues of the Great White Glow.

Find yourself a piece of white paper with nothing on it. A scrap will do or the back of the business card or a blank page in a book. Hold the white paper at a comfortable distance in front of you (6 to 16 inches may do). Notice its reflective quality and its degree of whiteness.

Close your eyes now and relax your arms. With your nose paint brush, paint yourself a white egg. This egg is sitting in the morning sunshine on a white lace doily that has been freshly laundered in

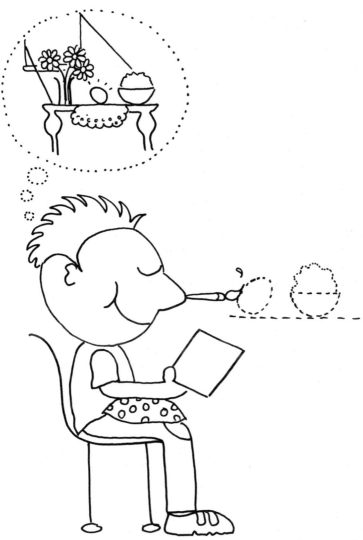

bleach. The white doily is resting on the top of a white-lacquered, round table. The sunshine is also shining on a milk glass vase filled with a crowd of white daisies. *Imagine* that you reach out your finger and touch the glowing whiteness of one daisy petal. A white soup bowl full of fresh snow appears. Then you pat the gleaming white egg, caress for a moment the texture of the lace, rub the sheen on the table, and taste the cool clean white snow. White is in your mind and imagination. Brilliant clear sunlit whiteness. As you savor this whiteness, allow your eyes to open and bring your white paper back to its former position in front of you. Scan it once more.

Is it whiter than before? This increase in your sensation of whiteness comes from the imagination of white. This permits you to: relax your vision, make a strong connection with the white, and increase the saccadic movement necessary for easy reading.

EYES AND THE PRINTED WORD

Reading is the act of moving the eyes and mind across language symbols and coming up with meaning. This act involves both the right and left hemispheres of the brain and a relaxed, dynamic visual style. Our left hemisphere attends to the sounds and the logic of the words. The right hemisphere maintains an awareness of the whole visual field, rhythm, and dramatic expression.

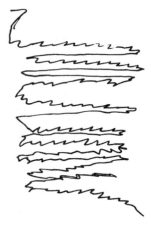

eye movements when reading (after Yarbus)

The eyes themselves leap about the words picking up the shapes to feed into both hemispheres of the brain and the visual cortex. The figure shows the way the eye moves when reading. There is a smooth side to side flow within which the eye jiggles around a letter using the smallest, quickest kinds of saccades. Alfred Yarbus, researcher of eye movements, found that in the reading of poetry, longer 'fixations' (the optometric term related to our 'nuclear vision') take place as the mind dwells on a particular thought/image. He draws the conclusion that the reading of printed text is therefore maintained entirely by the fovea centralis. Longer fixations suggest that the eye cooperates by shifting about a particular word while the mind fetches an image to go with it. No wonder the reading aloud of poetry has been found to be especially effective in turning on the whole brain. We get left brain words with right brain imagery.

On the other hand, studies of readers who stumble with awkwardness when reading aloud reveal that the eyes are pausing *too* long on a given word, almost like a visual stutter. The eyes are also staying with the words being spoken instead of running on ahead of the voice as happens when the reader is performing with elan, ease, and enjoyment. E.A. Taylor, who investigated a gifted reader, observed that the young man could read between 220 and 600 words per minute with total comprehension, picking up several words, or a whole phrase, with just one short saccadic fixation. The implication is that his left-and right-brains were phenomenally integrated and that his foveal vision was unusually agile.

THE WHITE WALTZ: DEVELOPING CLARITY WHEN READING

Place your magic paint brush on the end of your nose. The paint brush is attached to a huge bucket of the whitest paint you can imagine. Start at the top of a white card with black letters on it. (Use the letter card at the back of this book.) Paint the card white with big strokes, slapping the paint on. Your intention is to end up with the thickest, most brilliant white possible.

Paint white along the edges of the paper too. Here you may notice a narrow white stripe. This is the first indication of the presence

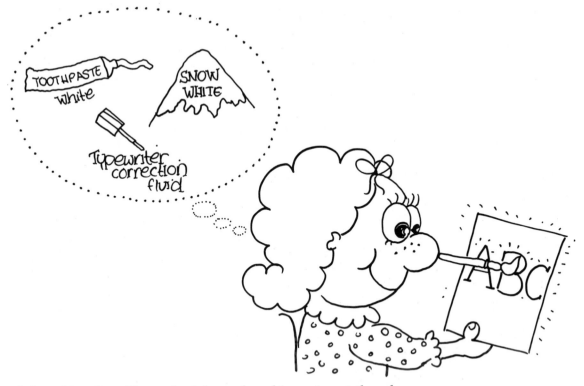

of the white glow. If you don't have the white stripe at the edge, *pretend* it is there and proceed with this activity. It may come later, quite spontaneously, if you open the 'pretend' door now.

Paint a white circle counterclockwise around one of the largest letters. Do you notice a white halo, aura, sheen, a white disc of light around the letter? This is the white glow. The white glow appears first along the edges of the paper then at the edges of letters. We preceive the black letters by the white light that forms the shape around them. The black ink of the letter sends nothing to our eyes. Black absorbs all the light. So if you are trying and straining to see the black letter you are acting under a common error. To try to see black is adding strain to a brain that's protesting, 'I'm not getting any input from this ink anyway. Why is the boss insisting that I make sense out of something that I don't have?'

The white background is the key to relaxed reading and finding the ability to clear up the perception of letters at any distance regardless of size. To do the White Waltz you:

1. Paint white around the letter.
2. Close your eyes and paint white around the letter. Emphasize the intensity of the white paint.
3. Open your eyes and paint white around the letter.

You may notice after opening your eyes that the white appears brighter and cleaner than before. If the white gets whiter, the black has to get blacker. The result is higher contrast between the ink and the paper. The letters will be clearer. Continue doing the three steps with the larger letters. Take your time. Rest by palming and sunning, stretching and yawning, often. Waltz your way with the paint brush, doing the three steps with progressively smaller letters.

The White Glow is at home everywhere on the page, around big letters and around the smallest letters. Therefore size makes no difference. You are able to see clearly tiny letters up close and big ones in the distance.

READING WITH THE GLOW

Now that you have begun tuning into the white spaces around letters and words, and have been flexing and toning your accommodation equipment with the paddle, it is time to adapt the White Glow to the process of reading. Find yourself some easy, pleasant reading material. Do a few minutes of sunning, a bit of palming and some tromboning. If your paddle is not close by, you can always use your hand. Sit comfortably for reading. The light is to come from behind or your side (the left side if you're right-handed, the right side if you are left-handed), or from straight above. Optimal indoor light would be at least a 100 watt bulb shining right on to your paper. You can also sit outdoors in full sunlight. If you are still building your tolerance to direct sunlight, sit in the shade.

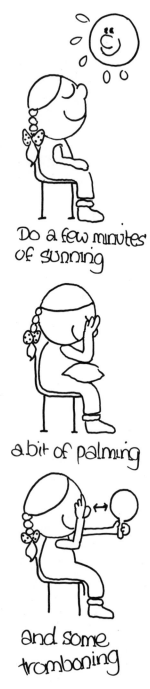

Do a few minutes of sunning

a bit of palming

and some tromboning

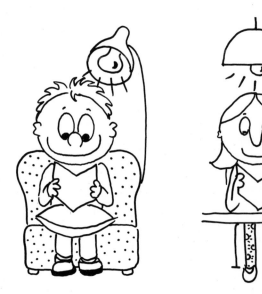

With your nose paint brush, begin to stroke white paint from left to right on top of the lines of print on your book. Blink easily. While painting, imagine that whiteness is alive and well in the back of your head. Your brain is familiar with the shapes of the letters

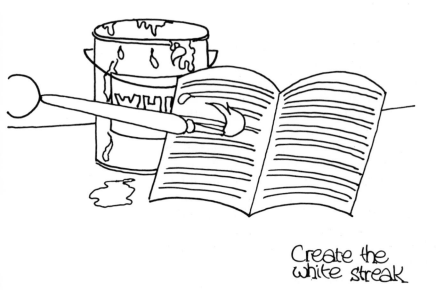

Create the
white streak

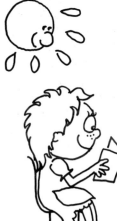

and the words. It will automatically produce the meaning of these configurations you have seen so many times before. Now is the time to accustom yourself to using the White Streak whenever you read. The White Streak is an offspring of the Great White Glow you danced round with in the White Waltz. The Glow turns from a circle around letters into a white streak that you paint through the lines of print. Do not worry about painting out the black letters. They will reassert themselves automatically.

Turn to the reading card in the back of this book. With your white nose paint brush stroke the white paint through the largest lines of print. Paint through the same line several times allowing the white ribbon or track of the White Glow to emerge. With continued easy breathing, blinking and painting move gradually along to the smaller and smaller lines of print. If you pause at the end of each paragraph to close you eyes and swish some white around the last word, you'll find your eyes returning right to the word imagined in a refreshed aura of whiteness.

Questions often arise about speed reading. The type of speed reading which eliminates subvocalization is the most compatible with the vision improvement games in this book. Subvocalizing means that you silently verbalize every word as you read. This slows down the act of reading considerably. It takes much longer to talk about something than it does to see it. The White Streak can aid in damping the subvocalizing habit as the verbal mind is occupied with the inner rhythmic thought 'white, white, white'. After a while this thought also fades away and you will be able to read with the white glowing streak for long periods of time, without fatigue.

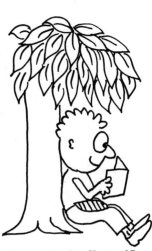

Clear Easy Reading Close and Far

WHITE GLOW GOES TO THE EYECHARTS

When you put letters on white paper and hang them in the distance they turn into eyecharts. The Great White Glow loves eyecharts. Waltzing on eyecharts will turn them into allies instead of enemies. For all eyecharts, makeshift or formal, do the White Waltz game just as you would for reading. It is helpful to put a picture of something with white in it nearby: the snowy moutains, white flowers, a white sailboat. Anything white in the vicinity will aid your imagination and keep your white aglow. Scatter white objects around the room or yard. A napkin, cotton balls, white cloth are suggestions. Play and make up your own white to white game, roaming from one white space to another. Sweep across the white of the eyechart with the same nonchalance you use when edging other white objects. Begin now to encircle the letters on the chart one at a time. Doing the three steps described in the White Waltz will enable the letters to pop out at you, clear as a bell. When you are satisfied with the whiteness of your paper, create flexibility of seeing by varying the distance of the card from your nose. Do this gradually. If the card is in your hand, move it 1 or 2 inches in or out. If the card or chart is in the distance, move it 1 or 2 feet to start. When the White Glow comes readily at one distance move the card again.

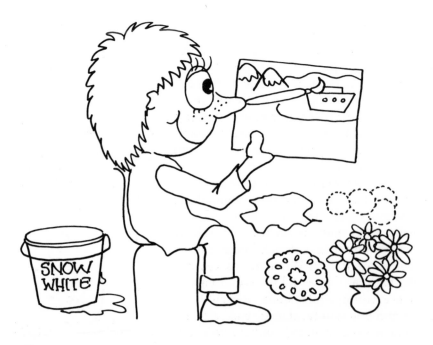

READING POSTURE AND STAMINA

To maintain the maximum flow of visual energy through your body and to keep both sides of your brain turned on, it is essential to keep your body channels open. Sitting to read is preferable to lying down. The latter can cramp the neck and restrict energy flow up the spine into the visual centres. If you like to read in bed put cushions behind you so you are sitting up. Place a pillow on your lap to bring the book up to the height where it is easy for your eyes to see without straining your neck. In this way you can keep your neck and head free to paint away with your white paint brush.

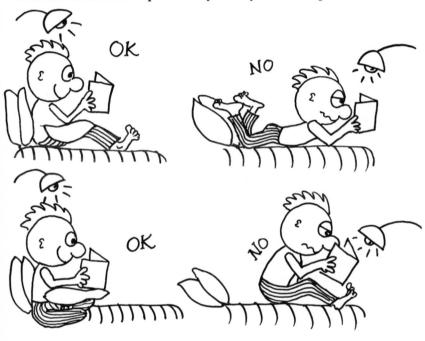

The placing of a cushion or pillow on your lap when reading will prevent arm fatigue, frozen head positioning and crossing of the legs, all which tend to deactivate part of your brain. Another reason for an upright and supported posture for reading is that it prevents the habit of covering one eye or tipping the head which you might do if lying on your side to read. This habit is often related to or could foster an imbalance between the two eyes.

Palming breaks are useful for studying as well as for clearing print. If you are reading to learn, pause at the end of each chapter and spend ten minutes palming, visualizing and playing with the content you gained from the chapter. When the verbal energy of reading is changed into visualizations, you have boosted your memory. Ask yourself, 'What is the main idea, of what I just received from this chapter (or page)?' Then tell yourself, 'I am going to put this idea into a visual image.' The memory courses that are popular in the world today are based on visualization techniques. To remember facts, you transform them into pictures, the more humorous the better (good humor has an 'in' with your memory banks). Draw and paint the visual images while you palm.

Take the white glow with you wherever you travel. Take it to the phone book, to dim restaurants, and on to computer screens. If the background color on your reading material is other than white, imagine that color.

May the glow be with you always.

May the glow go with you.

May the glow warm your heart.

May the thrill of the white find you at night.

P.S. Let the glow happen. When it happens. Until then *pretend*.

PALMING FOR WHITE

If you wish to increase your connection to the white space on a reading card, for playing with eye charts, or for relaxed reading, it is helpful to palm and visualize a white story such as this:

Once upon a time there was a little white mouse named Snowy. *Yawn*. Snowy had a long white tail and soft white fur, *Yawn*, little round white ears, a white nose and Snowy loved to *Yawn*. Everytime Snowy *Yawned*, white stuff would start to come down from the sky. Only the white stuff wasn't snow, it was cotton because Snowy lived in the cotton fields. *Yawn*. Every Easter Snowy would throw a party. *Yawn*. At the party he invited all the white animals into the cotton fields when the cotton was in full bloom. Huge white balls of cotton shone in the sunlight. *Yawn*. Snowy owned four thousand acres of cotton. He was into Agribiz. He always painted his tractors white and his cotton-picking machines as well. But before his machines moved into the field, he threw this wild white party, *Yawn*. He invited the white leghorn chickens. Of these his personal friends numbered fifty. Here they come. Fifty chickens. *Yawn*. Fifty white chickens. And they always dressed up for Snowy's parties in the cotton fields. Each chicken wears a white fancy lace costume, tiny white hat, with a small white apron made of fresh organza with eyelet lace along the edges. Pure white. If they got a smirch of anything on their costume they had to go back home and wash it out. Bleach it, starch it, wring it out, iron it, put it on again and return to the party. *Yawn*. As soon as the chickens got there, they would present their party-warming gifts, a beautiful pure white egg from each. Perfect white eggs. Fifty of them shining and gleaming in the sunlight. And the chickens are smiling. Snowy is so happy that he *Yawns and Yawns.* The cotton plants burst into bloom and cotton starts to fall over all the sleepy white partygoers.

The next animal Snowy invited to his party was the Great White Crocodile. Have you ever seen an albino crocodile? There's only one. In the whole world there's only one and it lives in Australia near Darwin. And it had to swim all the way across the Pacific around the bottom of South America (the natives thought it was a sailing ship) *Yawn* up the coast of Argentina and Brazil, through the turquoise lagoon waters of the Caribbean and up into the Mississippi Delta. Now it's ambling across the cotton fields to Snowy's party. The whitest crocodile you've ever seen. It crawls into the middle of the fifty leghorn chickens and smiles. There's also a white swan with a beeper who always comes to Snowy's parties. This swan flies from the northern snowfields of Canada. Look at the swan there in the snow taking off. Have you ever seen such a beautiful sight? A white swan taking off in the white snow? *Yawn.* You will know when it is airborne by the change in your breathing. It is glistening in the sunlight as it flies over Minnesota, over Tennessee, down into the South, drawn to the four thousand acres of white cotton. Gently it comes in for a landing, setting itself down into a pool that Snowy has provided for it, filled with white milk. SOOOOOOOOOwsheddddduddd into the milk. The white crocodile begins to swim anticlockwise in the white liquid. *Yawn. Yaaaaawwwwwwwwnnnnnnn.*

With the feeling and imagery of white still in the back of your mind, bring your hands away slowly and blink softly. Paint white over your book or eye chart while whiteness hovers in the back of your mind.

With the white alive and well in your mind, it will be clean and clear in your physical environment. Notice that the black letters stand out from the white on their own. They are proud to be associated with such astounding whiteness.

Chapter 15.

Supporting Children's Vision

The joy and openness of young eyes is always a pleasure and inspiration. The eyes of children candidly mirror the wonder and beauty of the world. Supporting and nurturing this unsullied organic responsiveness of beginning and growing vision is the theme of this chapter.

An explosion of growth and development takes place in the infant during the first year outside the womb. Dependent, cooing nurslings become mobile perceptive vocal somebodies. Innocent eyes have thoroughly tasted the world one at a time, then brought themselves together. Expanding brains have laid down cross-coordinating path ways for binocular vision both close and far. The one-year-old registers the doggie down the street and the bit of lint on your sleeve.

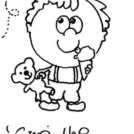

'Give the kid a carrot!'

Even by the end of the first astonishing year, a child's vision is by no means a finished product. The exploring and synthesizing of physical, mental and emotional patterns will continue for years before the visual system stabilizes into the flexible, keen perceptive and expressive faculty it is meant to be.

Rushing children prematurely into walking, into eating with utensils (a sign of solidified dominance meant to appear after age three) and other advanced behaviors can have the opposite effect to that desired by parents. It can result in a lack of integration and performance in school when the child is older. Dyslexia, crossed eyes, stuttering and lack of body coordination have been traced to interferences in the normal progression of neurological patterning. From sixteen weeks to six months our infants naturally express homolateral action of body, eyes, and ears. From six months to one year the mid-brain, the bridge between right and left hemispheres of the brain, is called into play through crawling. Walkers, playpens, tight clothing, even shoes and early coaxing into walking are potential impediments to this crucial cross-patterning stage. From three to five years, right or left hand dominance appears as the continuing

NATURALLY HOMOLATERAL INFANTS

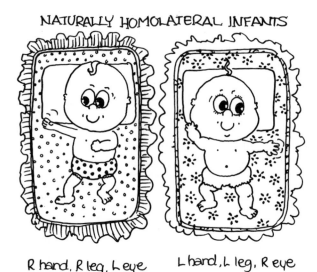

R hand, R leg, L eye   L hand, L leg, R eye

'The Creeper'
appears at 6 months
to 1 year. Eyes and
ears begin to act
together. Eye/hand
co ordination occurs

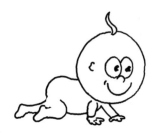

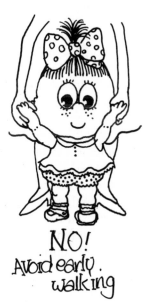

NO!
Avoid early.
walking

organization of body, mind, eyes, and cultural adaptations continues apace.

Never mind despairing if you've already used walkers, or tottled your child across the floor, or if there has been an illness or injury that slowed down your baby's performance through these stages. It is possible to retrace and reintroduce balancing actions at any time which will help recoordinate the system — through cross-crawl (chapter 12) for example and your consistent searching love.

Given some positive, knowledgeable, loving support by parents and teachers, maturing children always regulate themselves in the direction of health and balance. At natural vision centers, we have found that when parents have transmuted their fears, gained an understanding of the factors affecting their child's visual expression, and learned some appropriate games to play with their children, they are able to positively assist their child's eyesight.

EARLY CHILDHOOD INFLUENCES

Knowledge about children's vision is conspicuously lacking in the home and school. When something does go awry, parents are completely dependent on the opinions of whatever expert they take the child to. It behooves parents to request from doctors as much knowledge in this area as possible. A lot of new and old research on visual development is available, but mainly accessible only to professionals. In fact the work of some early researchers on children's visual and perceptual development is still extremely valuable. In the 1940s, Arnold Gesell, M.D. conducted a ten year study of children's vision at the Yale Clinic of Child Development. Darrel Boyd Harmon spent several years analysing the crucial effect that school environments have on children's vision and general well-being. We will use both Gesell's and Harmon's discoveries in findings ways to support optimum home experience for our children's vision.

It was long thought that newborn infants had little, if any, seeing capacity. Therefore early visual experiences were considered inconsequential and not influential in vision development. The glare and bright lights of delivery rooms could not therefore affect the neonate in any way. Stark white nurseries were thought hygienically optimal for infants who spent most of their time sleeping anyway. Caustic silver nitrate drops were routinely wiped through babies eyes and regarded as harmless.

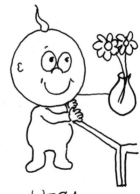

YES!
When they are
ready they will
go for it at just
the right point.
(walking
that is!)

Fortunately the increase of gentle birthing methods and pre-birth education for parents may begin to lower the incidence of vision imbalances due to rough deliveries and callous treatment of the newborn's perceptive faculties. Osteopaths and chiropractors both have methods for altering the ill effects of forceps used in deliveries, or from early accidents. Re-aligning the bones of the neck and skull and adjusting the spine have made huge differences in childhood astigmatism and visual uncoordination.

Now we learn that babies are far more visually sensitive, perceptive, and advanced at birth than was ever suspected. In 1982 in a conference in New York, researchers on cognitive psychology, brain development, vision, hearing, anthropology, and paediatrics met to discuss just what the infants of the world are seeing. Some psychologists devised ways to ask the babies themselves. Babies, they learned, are able to track a geometric shape on the day they are born. As soon as an hour after birth some newborns are imitating visual facial movements as complex as sticking out the tongue. Moving right along, these amazing infants are able to tell the difference between colours at three months. The adaptable visual faculties continue to concentrate and express energy in a maturing process for years to come. In his book *Vision, Its Development in Infant and Child*, Arnold Gesell reports to us that: 'During the first decade of life the components of the entire visual-motor system undergo ceaseless organization and reorganization, adapting not only to cultural demands but even more to the structural changes within the organism [child] itself. General body posture, lying, crawling, standing, sitting, squatting, squirming, jumping, are all accompanied by increasingly refined eye-hand coordination mediated through the musculature.'

THE AMBLYOPIA QUESTION

Amblyopia means lower vision when there is no observable cause (such as refractive errors). According to a leaflet put out by the California Optometric Association, amblyopia is 'very common'. Sometimes amblyopia follows in the wake of squint. One prevailing theory is that if a squint (turned eye) has developed the baby or child sees double. To overcome this, nature, via the brain, psychologically 'suppresses' the vision of the deviating eye and amblyopia results. The cause of this condition is a mystery to doctors. They speculate that the trouble lies in 'a lack of development somewhere along the optic nerve or in the brain centre'. Developmental optometrists recommend early consultation with a vision therapist (themselves) so that a patch, vision exercises or lenses can be prescribed.

In *Ophthalmology Made Ridiculously Simple*, the author states that amblyopia is a tiny defect in the wiring of the eye to the brain that comes from disuse of one eye early in life, 'usually before the age of seven'. The prediction is that if glasses are not prescribed quickly the child will suffer irreversible lack of sight in that eye. The response of correcting faulty vision with glasses does not do anything for amblyopic eyes after the age of seven according to this theory. If the child's eye turns in the wrong direction medical doctors often recommend surgery purely for cosmetic reasons. After surgery the child still does not necessarily obtain binocular vision. Vision therapists on the other hand insist that surgery is usually unnecessary.

If your child has an eye that is straying and you visit an ophthalmologist, he/she may say, 'We must operate immediately or the eye that is turning will become amblyopic.' With such operations, there is no guarantee that function will return to that eye, although it sometimes does when followed by vision therapy. However, vision therapists whose equipment is limited to machines, eye patches, glasses and exercises that require a more mature mind to do them, have little to offer parents of children under a year old. Sometimes children have numerous operations, their developing bodies being subjected several times to the toxicity of anaesthesia and the trauma of surgery. Scar tissue is formed on the muscles of the eye and usually glasses must still be worn. The effective work done with the thousands of squinting babies and children by the Corbett-Bates teachers in their homes during the 1930s through 1950s went ignored or snubbed by all the professional eye care groups.

Go for another opinion if you are in conflict about operating on a child with a wandering or turning eye. One Australian ophthalmologist gave a mother-client a dour reprimand, 'Stop mucking about. Operate now or you will be responsible for your baby going blind.' The baby was three months old. The mother took the child to another eye doctor, who said 'This child doesn't need an operation. It is normal for babies of his age to have wandering eyes.' I understand where the first opinion is coming from. Research does show that babies suddenly have depth perception, an indication of fusion, at around four months and it appears to be solidified at

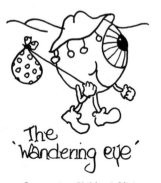

The 'wandering eye'

Supporting Children's Vision

five months. Yet I've seen adults who did not have binocularity (fusion) for years develop it as a result of a self-help vision program.

My response to calls for guidance in this area is to recommend that you make your judgement based on your knowledge, your motivation to do what you are able at home, and after weighing the opinions of the least two different doctors. It is especially important to release the immediate mental and emotional stress so that you are able to make a clear decision. If the child has such severe blur that only glasses will give him or her immediate relief, then use them and begin integrating the natural vision activities while your eye doctor periodically checks the child's progress. Fear is the main motive that causes nervous parents to force children into wearing glasses. Fear is fostered by patronizing doctors, concerned teachers at school and anxiety that the child will not come up to snuff academically. Fear has the interesting knack of actualizing that which it predicts. Release fear by using the emotional holding points on your forehead as on page 118. Ask lots of questions and trust your own decisions.

THE NATURAL VISION PATH FOR LITTLE ONES

The parents who have come to me asking for something they could do at home for their children's vision are 90 per cent of the time in a state of extreme 'switched off' tension. The mothers, particularly, feel inadequate. They have been intimidated in doctors' offices and feel guilty because their child did not turn out right. Clearing these feelings is important for a home environment conducive to vision change, and also for maintaining normal vision. Keep these thoughts in mind and heart:

1. Children are responsive to love (so are parents!!!).
2. Love is the strongest healer and the greatest relaxant.
3. When your mind is at ease, you will be able to find the information that is right for you in regard to your child's vision.
4. Any challenges that arise in yourself or your child are opportunities for you both to benefit even though it may not appear so at the moment.
5. The visual system, when given a naturalistic supportive environment, will tend to right itself.
6. Vision is an innate function which grows, develops, and adapts to both internal body changes and external environments.
7. Teach your child seeing the way you teach him/her to talk. Vision is best encouraged through play with tiny bits here

and there scattered throughout the day. Integrate little games into the rhythms of your practical and loving interaction.

8. Visual habits are imitated just as are ways of walking and talking. If you, the parent, improve your visual habits, your child will do so without a word from you. Sometimes mothers sporting a pair of thick glasses, turned down mouth and tight shoulders, bring their children to us saying, 'Oh, no, I don't want to join a class. It is too late for me. I just don't want my son (or daughter) to have to wear glasses.' Mom will be a non-participant and play the role of disciplinarian instead. 'Have you practised your eye exercises yet?' will echo through the house. All the fun, sharing, and communication is gone. If mom, dad, grandparents, or friends play the games the children will join in, just as they did with speaking, rattling pots and pans, building with hammer and saw, etc.

9. Meet the children in their world. This is a challenging thing to do but entirely possible if you simply imagine being a child again yourself. Let go of dignity and get down on the floor with the little ones to play vision games. You too will become relaxed and energized, young again.

10. Use the ideas and activities that follow freely. As you expand and express, variations on the themes will arise from the joy shared by you and your children.

ACTIVITIES FROM BIRTH TO ONE MONTH OLD INFANTS

Take him out of his plastic box and hold him close to your heartbeat. Lay him on your tummy when you rest. The important things now are warmth, satisfaction and light. Give him the rhythmical

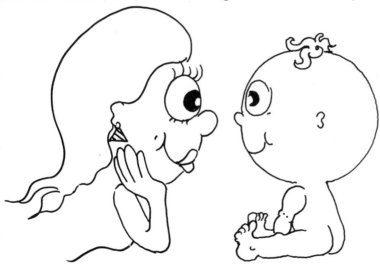

experiences he had in the womb such as humming, cooing, sway-ing. Smiling, friendly faces coming in close for a nuzzle are wonder-ful to stimulate vision and give love and warmth. Bring large, brightly colored objects within close range to satisfy his visual interest. When holding and breastfeeding the baby, he/she is automatically switch-ed from side to side. Each eye is then stimulated in turn. If bottle feeding, be sure to do this as well. One eye will become dominant later on, yet we don't want to neglect the other eye which is meant to start fusing with the 'leader' eye at around two to four months.

ACTIVITIES FOR ONE TO FOUR MONTH OLD INFANTS

To encourage saccadic movement and the ability to track, hand play activities such as snapping fingers, making hand figures or pat-a-cake. Sing along with this game:

PAT-A-CAKE
Pat-a-cake, pat-a-cake, baker's table,
Bake me a cake as fast as you're able
Roll it and pat it, and mark it with a 'B',
Put it in the oven for baby and me.

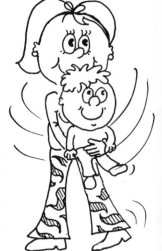

Take brightly colored balls of yarn and twirl them. Put a bob-bing creature in front of your baby. Do the Dance of the Eaglet.

Hold the infant in your arms so that the child is facing outward. Sway your baby from side to side or turn pivoting on your toes so that the world slides gently past both of you. If you are wearing glasses, take them off. You and the kid are in this together. The Eaglet Swing can be done to music, in front of a mirror or outdoors in pleasant surroundings (not too noisy please). Hum, sing, croon, babble, yawn, make silly sounds together. This activity can be done with tiny babies up until the time they are too heavy to hold. Sometimes the infant will fall asleep from the soothing quality of the motion. This could become a favorite routine for both of you. If the child is older and gets restless, put him/her down. The vision games are never meant to be restrictive or unpleasant.

ACTIVITIES FOR FOUR TO EIGHT MONTH OLD INFANTS

Continue to offer visually intriguing objects which can be sent roll-ing across the floor as distance perception expands. Finger and toe play is excellent whilst singing this classic:

THIS LITTLE PIG
This little pig went to market, this little pig stayed home.
This little pig had nice roast beef, this little pig had none.
But this little pig cried, 'Wee, wee, wee, wee' all the way home.

With your fingers, creep from toe to chin singing little Arabella
Millar (to the tune of Twinkle, Twinkle, Little Star):

LITTLE ARABELLA MILLAR
Little Arabella Millar found a woolly caterpillar.
First it crawled upon her mother, then upon her baby brother;
All said, 'Arabella Millar, take away that caterpillar.'

If an eye is turning in or out, or up or down, cover the child's
other eye briefly with your hand while you sing. Your fingers tickling
skin will coax the eye in the direction you want to see it go. This
is the time of the eye, hand, and mouth concerto. Present a palatable
object. You'll get a total centering of attention with the eyes, body
and gaze. Sometime during this time period, that object will be
grasped and sent directly to the mouth. Gesell considered mouthing
to be a way of perceiving space. Never mind if the child's attention
dissolves suddenly. It is meant to. Organic growth involves a cyclic
consolidation and then disorganization to allow the advent of new
input through nerves, eyes, and motor actions. The eyes fluctuate
through the refractive error states. A seven and a half month old
infant was observed by retinoscopy (the objective examination of
the eye) while sitting on his mother's lap. The researchers waved
a rattle at a 15 feet distance. The child's eye sought the toy showing
a reflexic 'with' hyperopic response. When its attention relaxed with
identification of the rattle, the eyes went into an 'against' myopic
reflexic response. This plus and minus, give and take fluctuation in
the child's vision will continue through the ensuing years. It corresponds to the 'taking in' and 'giving out' processes. Introjection,
identification, grasping of ideas/shapes in space, reciprocates with
projection outward, pointing, extending oneself into the environment.

Palming can become a lifelong habit for anyone, including your
infant. If you begin covering the child's eyes with your hands for short
periods early on, the child will accept palming as a natural activity.
This later leads to peek-a-boo games where the child covers his/her
own eyes. Use finger puppets (or just a spoon) to favor a direction
if called for to encourage an eye to go out or in. Eventually bedtime
stories will be listened to while everyone is palming. Continue pat-a-
cake with the hands or feet. Trombone toys in and out briefly then
place them into the baby's hands. Stimulating toys could include baby-
safe chewable stuffed animals, chimes, rattles, and crib gyms. Bedtime is a merry time with endless sociable variations of seeing,
touching, grasping, twisting, mouthing.

'peek-a-boo'
games

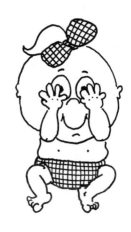

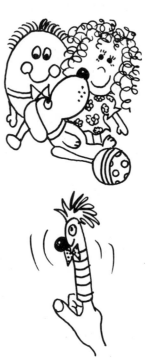

Supporting Children's Vision

ACTIVITIES FOR EIGHT TO TWELVE MONTH OLD INFANTS

Play with things that go high in space encouraging flexing of the upper body and back of the neck. Encourage crawling and pushing through 'tunnels' of cushions and chairs. This helps to coordinate upper and lower brains. Let the children walk when *they* are ready. Tracking is stimulated by having the child watch bigger folks playing catch or rolling a ball. Use repetitive nursery games to stimulate visual memory such as 'Where is sister? Where is Dad?' Little fingers want to explore and the kitchen provides a treasury of plastic nesting 'boxes'. Notice how your baby blinks when banging spoons on pots or pounding on something. Keep a kitchen drawer full of 'exploitables'.

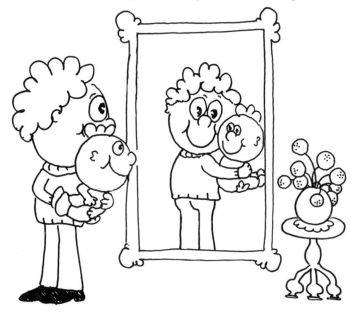

Spend time infront of the mirror together

Games which encourage little fingers to find things inside other things such as a cork in a cup or an apple under a dishtowel are fascinating. Play a game where you point to something and the baby crawls to touch it. Tickles and hiding under the blankets of the bed playing 'Pop Goes the Weasel' promotes a flow of laughter. Become kinetic yourself. Dance while swinging. Spend time in front of the mirror together. Do directional swinging. A backward glance outward over the shoulder into the mirror will help bring a turned-in eye outward. Sing blinking songs in which you substitute the word 'blink' for the ordinary words. When you sing 'blink', everyone's eyes blink.

A moderate amount of light is essential for the infant's health and visual growth. Babies need ultraviolet on their skin to develop vitamin D and for proper pituitary stimulation. Take baby for walks in a backpack or stroller and go out on treasure hunts in the grass to provide sunlight and fresh air. Sun yourself and children will follow. Eventually a one year old child may be closing his/her eyes and circling the sun in imitation of you.

ACTIVITIES FOR ONE TO FOUR YEAR OLDS

Continue with the integrative psycho-physical action of crawling. This crossing movement can be done on the back with lots of tickles and hugs. It now moves into being a dance form with hopping and jigging to lively music. Combine the cross-crawling with lots of 'follow the leader' games. More complex toys appear that can be dragged, pushed, climbed on. For three and four-year olds, provide a private box full of buttons, bits of cloth, stones, bright odds and ends for fingers to feel and eyes to 'touch' simultaneously.

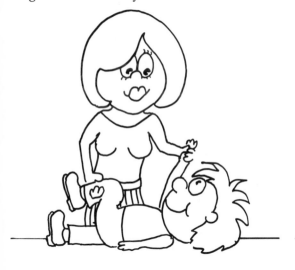
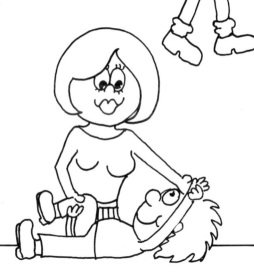

Simple sound-makers like gongs, triangles, drums, tambourines, and more can be played with. Hide behind a chair and make a beep or thump to call forth sound location followed by a visual revelation.

For palming, mutually view a simple object, then palm and imagine it 'inside your head' for a few seconds. *See!* is the big word. See mirrors, thunderclouds, the blender. Imitate the sounds of objects. Play 'Where are your eyes?' and 'Where are my eyes?' Provide huge building blocks or stack pillows on top of pillows. Provide books with pictures in them and areas for scribbling.

Acting and theatre becomes a thrilling way to encourage imagination through the body. Act out the farmer and the pig, the mailman and the child, the tree and the bird. Reverse roles. Have your child massage you or tell you a story while you palm.

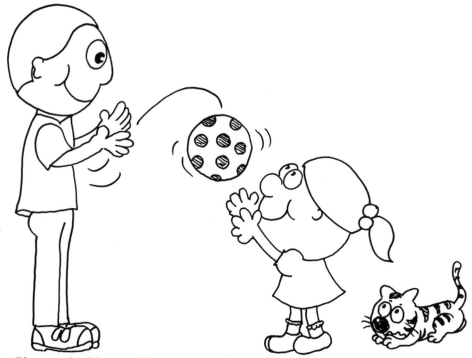

Play catch. Obtain different size balls in various bright colors. Have your child pick one and make friends with it, sniff it, talk with it. You pick one too. Connect your noses with your balls so that wherever they go your noses follow. Hold the ball in your hand and circle it counterclockwise with your nose. Toss it to your small companion with exhalation, a sound, Hahaaaaaaah. When the ball meets her hands, she circles it with her nose (puts her mark on it) and tosses it back to you. Exchange balls. If you are playing with a tiny tot, this game may stay on the floor. If you're playing with a bigger tot who can stand and catch, start the game very close. With success, move gradually farther away. The ball disappears into a basket or behind a chair or bush to re-emerge and twinkle through the air. Use a lot of spontaneous fantasies, whimsy, breathing, giggles and rowdiness.

The four year olds are ready for vision excursions into the big (right-brain) world. The sky, the ocean, visiting a park or the neighbors are all great. Go out for your adventure, then return and palm to respond to the questions stimulated from your outing such as, 'What does the ocean look, taste, smell or feel like?'

ACTIVITIES FOR FIVE TO SEVEN YEAR OLDS

To satisfy the eager left-brain of the five year old, do matching games such as matching a leaf on the ground to a leaf on a tree, or a

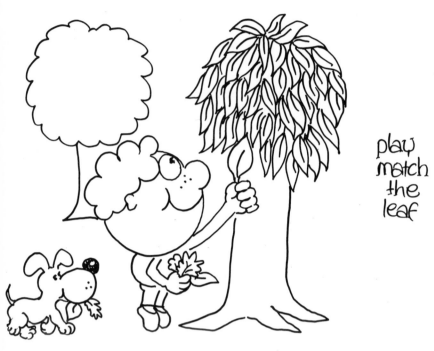

play
match
the
leaf

color in the hand found again at increasingly further distances by scanning with the nose. Lotto games done with or without patching will keep the attention flowing as the mind sorts and categorizes. The Gate from chapter 13 becomes a magic trick. Have the child observe how each side of the Gate appears and disappears as alternate eyes are covered. The child can play with the Gate like a trombone, swinging with it and noticing the trees sliding past. During palming activities, help the child to visualize going to Africa, or to the zoo to watch how the animals yawn. Go together to the high seas and visit a pirate with patching.

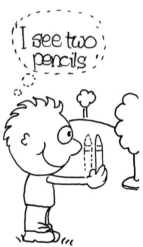

Movement activities like the Bird Dance and full-bodied Near-Fars swings are good for the five year old. Include a lot of movement to music: Big Band music and 1950s rock and roll call out the little 'boppers'. Do cross-crawl activities while lying on the back, standing and walking around the room. Become an animal. Have him/her choose an animal that walks on all fours and let the animal crawl around the room. Organize cross-crawl relay races. If possible, obtain a mini trampoline. The child plays sketching and visualizing games while experiencing weightlessness on the trampoline. Adapt the ancient game of hopscotch to patching. To loosen tight shoulders and neck muscles, give the child a gentle massage. Get mini authoritarians to roll about on the floor, do somersaults, and crow like Peter Pan to loosen up grim postures.

With six years olds, do the fusion Gate and the bead games to help with eye-hand-mind coordination through their continuing cycles of mental and emotional rearrangments. Palm with stories involving color and the body. Examples might include: turning into blue people, tree people, yawning golden tigers, or basking green turtles. Introduce new names for colors such as apple, blood, tomato, carnation red. Go on vision walks in the neighborhood with these colors in the back of your minds looking for examples which can later be used in visualizing. Read and write poetry together. Illustrate your original creations or the retelling of old familiar poems. It is a perfect time for Mr Squiggle to appear. Mr Squiggle is a well-known Australian television star whose nose is a pencil with which he draws things in two dimensions. His drawings then become three dimensional, 'real', useable, even edible.

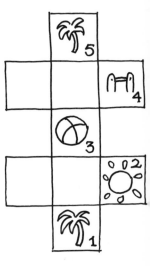

ACTIVITIES FOR EIGHT TO TEN YEAR OLDS

Tell a lot of jokes, have puppet shows (with patches) and play board games. The nose feather brushes across chess, checkers and monopoly boards. Palm and visualize money, gold coins, investments. Do counting or multiplication tables using imagery. For example, imagine two squirrels running to join two other squirrels on a log.

Stories told in a palming circle are great fun. To instigate a palming circle, lie down in the fresh green grass of your living room

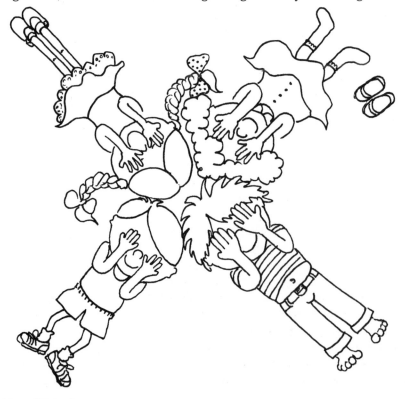

1. Here we palm to start the game
2. Here we sun our eyes
3. Here we play catch
4. Here we see the 'gate'
5. And we palm again to end the game

floor or in the sweet smelling hay mound on your bed. Invite some other people or just yourself. Cup your hands a bit and place them over your eyes so that light is closed out. Say thank you to your hands for their warmth and energy which are now flowing into your eyes and brain. Someone begins a story. Start with a character you are familiar with. Describe this character in detail (color, size, clothes, and personality). Take this character off on an adventure. At a crucial moment, pass the story on to someone else. The story need not make sense, what is important is that it produces images in the mind. Give people sounds, tastes, textures and some visual surprises. Here's our example from three nine year olds:

First Person: Rap, Rap, Rap, I hear a knocking on my door. I'm opening my door and there stands Miss Piggy. She is wearing an emerald green evening dress and a huge flashing diamond ring on her little pink pinky. On her head is a round red hat with one big yellow feather sticking out of it. She's winking a cute blue eye at me, grabbing my hand and pulling me into a . . .

Second Person: Little blue go-cart. We're tearing down the street toward the woods. We're bumping, bumping, bumping all the way past McDonalds and past two tall giraffes that are strolling down the street. Now we're entering the shadowy woods and driving our blue go-cart right inside a big oak tree. There are purple stairs inside the tree. It smells like turpentine. We're starting to climb the stairs . . .

Third Person: Suddenly, the big oak tree disappears. We're in mid-air and Miss Piggy says, 'goodbye'. She disappears, pouf, and is replaced by a giant vase of flowers made of pink pinkies, with diamond rings on them. The pinkies are singing 'Reach Out, Reach Out and Touch Someone'. The vase disappears. Now I'm hanging between a cloud of popcorn and a sun made of swiss cheese. I feel hungry so I swim through the sky toward the popcorn cloud. But I'm not getting anywhere. I start falling and land on another pop-corn cloud. I look down at my body and don't see anything although I can still feel myself. Then Daffy Duck appears and says . . .

You can also set up bowling, croquet or badminton games. On the writing board or on paper make lots of 'abstract' art starting with lazy eights, spirals, and mandalas as in chapter 9. Pretend you're yawning animals: a roaring lion, a hazy hippopotamus, an archaic alligator, a monstrous monkey (monkeys bang on their chests when yawning). Yawn as loud as possible. See who can yawn the loudest.

Sketch animal pictures in space with the nose pencil. Become a musical instrument with tromboning, making the sounds of various instruments. Pretend you are all part of an orchestra as it tunes up. Patch for pirate treasure hunts and do cross-crawl during the search. Play a lot of ball, catching at different distances and shooting baskets. Move the basket to different positions so the eyes move

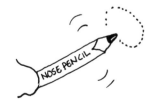

Supporting Children's Vision

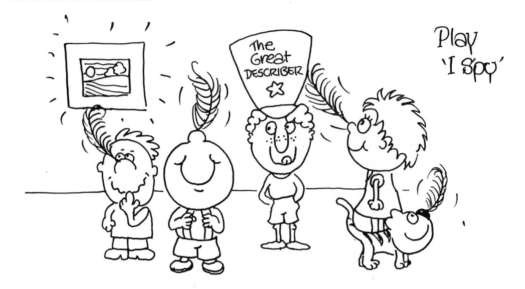

in all directions. Play I Spy. I Spy is an excellent nuclear vision game. It encourages the mind and eyes to play together. Based on the concept that what you're thinking/imaging is what you see, it helps develop visual alertness. Have everyone close their eyes, except the person who is the Great Describer. The Great Describer describes in color and detail an observable object without naming that object. The Great Describer draws upon her/his powers of description giving as many clues as possible, such as size, temperature, textures, etc. During this description, the other players, the 'Feather Dusters', visualize whatever images may be coming to them. When the great describer is finished with the description, all the players open their eyes and begin to dust the room with long fluffy feathers attached to the ends of their noses. Players wait for the object to 'pop out' or 'come alive', then sing out its name with 'I spy ....'. The first Feather Duster to call out the right object then becomes the next great describer.

In response to the frequently asked question, 'What about television?', I offer these questions for all parents to consider: Are the children being 'captured' by the television so that their creative energies are being nullified by the mass media? Or are they being inspired to make up their own TV programs, writing their own scripts and commercials? Is their sedentary activity balanced with bike-riding, tree-climbing, swimming or other physical activities? Are they staring into TV, books, or space most of the time? If you do see your child's energy being syphoned off into de-energizing habits that are overly passive, it is important that you respond not by chiding or nudging but by becoming active yourself in some way that will motivate and inspire the child. Go for walks, play together, even cleaning house can turn into a fiesta. What about video games? Playing video games at home draws forth from the child the ability to coordinate the hands and the eyes while maintaining movement, nuclear vision and visual flexibility. If these skills are translated to the world at large then the games are beneficial.

THE CLASSROOM AS A HAZARD

Starting in the 1940s, Darell Boyd Harmon commenced a long-range study of 4,000 schoolroom environments and their effects on the over all health and development of the 160,000 children who sat in them. Fifty-two per cent of these children left elementary school with obvious preventable problems in the areas of vision, posture, nutrition, infections, and behavior. A direct correlation was drawn between these health disorders and the environmental factors of restraining seating equipment and improper lighting.

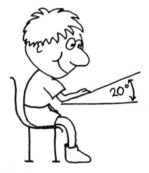

Both feet are planted on the floor, not crossed, thrust forward or back.

Harmon found that individual desks with tilting tops for reading and writing allowed a child freedom of movement in several directions (as opposed to large flat top tables where several children sit together). The appropriate angular relationships to provide for balanced posture was determined to be a tilt of 20° from the horizontal. This posture is optimal for close visual activities, lung expansion, uncompressed digestion and untwisted spines.

Lighting is equally important in relieving children of schoolroom stress. Diffused, even illumination that comes from the side without glaring into the child's eyes is imperative. In addition, we've learned that if we want to center our mind on a particular topic, we don't want our visual attention pulled away by highly contrasting edges in the periphery of our visual field. This is why dark brown desk tops were replaced by natural wood finish. The eyes are then able to shift saccadically around the words or letters on the white sheet of paper without being distracted by the high contrast between the white paper and the dark brown desk top. This same reasoning prompted the changeover from high contrast blackboards to the matte yellow-green boards in use today as these produce less subliminal distraction away from desk tasks or demonstrating teachers. The color yellow-green is used because the eye at rest sees the yellow-green part of the spectrum without undue accommodation. Unlike the camera, the human eye is not corrected for the fact that the seven spectral colors have differing wavelengths. Therefore, different colors focus themselves at different points along the optical axis. Harmon says 'The eye is myopic for radiation shorter than yellow-green and far-sighted for radiation, or color, longer than yellow-green — *a situation which in action it attempts to overcome*' (author's emphasis). The effort made by the eye/mind in reducing the adverse effects of distractive colors in classrooms is accomplished by freezing into a myopic or hyperopic adjustment. The optical

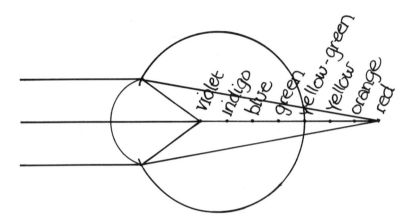

illusions and apparent alterations of size of objects due to the use
of warm versus cool colors and changes in background color was
studied by Dr Samuel Renshaw at Ohio State University in 1948-49.
He found that the apparent size of objects varied from 37 to 67 per
cent. These shifts and distortions due to environmental colors and
lighting can easily cause an adaptive shift in a child's eye of at least
one half a diopter, the level at which corrective glasses are deemed
necessary. For optimum use of colors to foster rather than hinder vision, background colors are to be 'greyed'. The teaching materials
themselves are to have full color value and be 'glowing' so that they
'pop out' of the secondary background. As a result of incorporating
these principles into schools, Harmon's group found that visual dif-
ficulties for 1,764 children dropped from 53 to 18.6 per cent in six
months, nutritional problems fell from 71 to 37 per cent and chronic
fatigue went from 21 to 7 per cent. As new schoolrooms are built,
Harmon's influence has been felt and utilized to some extent. These
crucial ideas concerning furniture, posture, lighting and color usage
could be employed in homes and offices as well.

If we pay attention to lighting, desk design, and decor in schools,
will our children then emerge from the other end of the system
clear-eyed, inspired, and ready to 'take on the world'? Possibly not,
for the external forces bearing on the children constitute only half
of the picture. Raymond Gottlieb, a behavioral optometrist created
the Eye Gym in Los Angeles. Dr Gottlieb graciously demonstrated
his eclectic and innovative ideas for enhancing children's vision for
my Natural Vision instructor training groups. Dr Gottlieb commented
on the link between schooling and eyesight in the *Brain-Mind Bulletin*.
'The tension generated by current methods of education is a major
cause of nearsightedness (myopia) and other visual problems. In

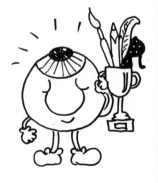

school, we are taught to squeeze and hold on to information, to be sure we've "got it" rather than let it come to us'.

Imagine how often the combination of internal personal and external environmental factors will bring a child to the point of wearing glasses. Allison Fuller, a Natural Vision instructor in Pasadena, California, told me that her daughter went into glasses at the age of fifteen because she couldn't see the board in calculus class. 'She could have been two inches away and blurred those numbers. Math was not her forte. She was taking it solely to prove to her father that she was smart enough.'

The tension is comprehensive — emotional, mental, and physical, and results in a lack of confidence in self (self love). Gottlieb states: 'Our perceptual abilities function best when we know that we can handle the environment successfully. But if we expect the environment to overwhelm us, our sensory integration will fragment and our perceptual fields will shrink.'

In other words, rather than sacrificing children's enthusiasm to prestige and propriety we might more avidly support their creative expressions in loving 'switched on' environments. Then we may all become more 'bright-eyed and bushy-tailed'.

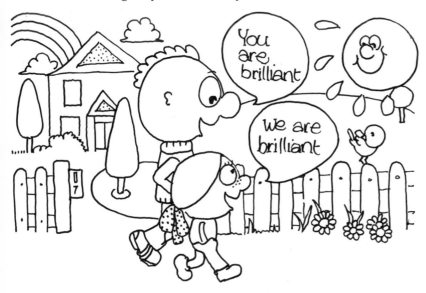

Chapter 16.

Guiding Yourself into Seeing

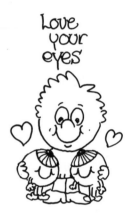

By now you've realized the advantages of approaching eyes with loving tenderness and appreciation. Our precious visual system provides 80 per cent of the brain's total input. You have, therefore, an opportunity to affect a major part of your life. The information you require is in your hands. Mother Nature provides the materials — The leaves on the trees, the architecture of cities and villages, the faces of people are stimuli to bring the knowledge out of this book and into your life.

Collect images and memories when you go on outings and vacations. Bring the flowers from the gardens into the office. Take the near-far swing (page 53) and the red ball (page 65) with you on trips. Carry your magic pencil, paint brush, and feather in your pocket. Freely adapt any and all of the ideas in this book to your own lifestyle. Add some, eliminate others that don't fit your ways at this time. Personally experimenting and creating your own variations on the principles you've learned is essential for a lasting improvement in seeing. This action will, in turn, lead you to new discoveries about yourself.

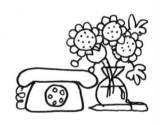

We're not going to throw the clock out the window or float off into space when improving vision naturally. It's fully integrated total-brain expression that we desire — a useful blend of relaxation and accomplishment. The following program suggestions are guidelines for you to experiment with. First we assure ourselves that the basics — movement, imaging and sunning are ongoing themes in your life. Then we'll add in the specialty items such as fusion and patching. Our final integration games take clarity to the eyecharts. At the end of this chapter I'd like you to entertain some ideas about diet and eye 'dis-ease'.

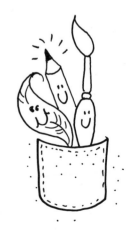

DEFINING YOUR OWN PROGRAM

A defined plan that explicitly pins down the activity, the length of time and when it's to be done is pleasing to some people. This kind of mapping will keep left-brain dominant people calm. It may also anchor the right-brain types who tend to scatter in all directions without a list to ground them. We will soften the severity of the grid plan by using a pictographic code as follows. I'm imagining that this translation of verbal instructions into images will be an agreeable way for you to adopt the vision themes into your life. The Code:

	Edging, sketching, constant movement
	Sunning
	Palming and Visualizing
	Near-Far Swings
	The Bird Dance
	Nuclear Vision activities
	Cross-crawl
	Patching
	The Bead Game
	The Great White Glow
	The Painting Game
	Yawning
	Transforming emotions
	Tromboning
	Mandala

Add your own pictographs:

Two areas may be considered to help set up a program on your chart. The first is the label that has been placed over the status of your vision. Are you myopic, hyperopic, or presbyopic? (be sure to differentiate between the last two.) Quiz your eye practitioner about it if you are not sure about 'your' label.

The second area is totally your option. What parts of yourself or your sight would you like to spruce up? Depending on your answer to that question, the appropriate games are added to your chart.

Here is an Activity Reference Chart. If you are, for example, myopic and have a wandering eye as well, pull the corresponding pictographs from the reference chart and draw them on the empty grid in the sequence you prefer.

ACTIVITY REFERENCE CHART

For Myopia Do							
For Hyperopia Do							
For Astigmatism Do							
For Presbyopia Do							
To Strengthen Fusion Do		color plate 4					
For Wandering Eye(s) Do							
To Remove Emotional Blocks							
To Develop Near Acuity				color plate 3			
To Develop Far Acuity							
To Develop Imagery							
To 'Switch On'							
To Nurture Vision Generally							
For Amblyopia Do							
To Develop Reading							

Natural Vision Improvement

An example; You are myopic, want to develop better fusion and
you know that body movement enlivens your life.

							Where	Time	When
My label is:	myopic	☼						10 min	after breakfast
		⟋						all the time	→
		🌴					🧎	whenever	after each chapter
		↶					🚪🔑	30 times	when I go to the post box
I want to develop:	fusion clear flashes	✳						10 mins	only on Sunday
		🎨						20 mins	every saturday P.M.
for fun I will	Dance	✕	♪	🍃				through many yawns	before bed

This empty grid is for you to fill in as you please from the
foregoing Activity Reference Chart.

A CIRCULAR PLAN

Stop, before you run away from the boxy chart above. Those of you who 'freak out' at organized disciplined plans, consider a circular approach. On the deepest level, we know that our life and being are pulsating in the rhythms of circles and spirals. To please your spatial, right-brain nature design yourself a mandala-like image that coordinates your daily cycles and the vision improvement games. Sit down for a moment and visualize yourself arising, bathing, eating, working. Now picture the vision activities you would like to 'hook up' to those daily actions. Sketch yourself (don't be shy) in action and then add the vision pictographs to the cycle.

An example of a circular plan: I like to palm in the morning before I get out of bed. I'll sun on the way to my car. I'll do cross-crawl before sitting down at my desk at work. Near-far swings I can do out in the park while eating lunch. I'll do my tromboning as I organize my papers before leaving work. After dinner I'll play with the white glow under my new lamp. Back to palming again when I lie down to dream.

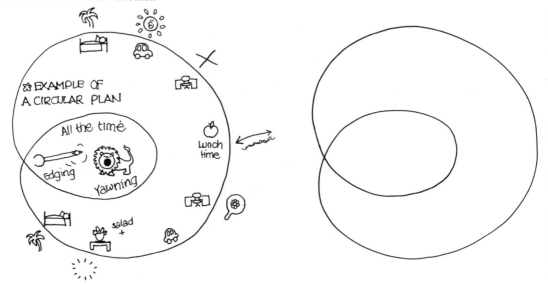

CLARITY GOES TO THE EYECHARTS

Imagine that I am with you on a sunny balmy day. We stroll into the garden or on to a hill after a lunch of salad with sprouts. We put on our nose pencils and sketch the landscape for a while, communing with the sky and the spirit of seeing. We've brought along a photograph (the cover of this book perhaps). Together with all good will, and the reverberating aliveness of all those seers who went before us, we take the following steps:

    1. Hold the photo where you see best. Scan back and forth

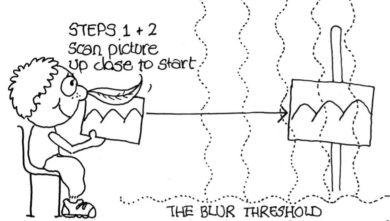

STEPS 1 + 2
Scan picture
up close to start

THE BLUR THRESHOLD

STEP 3
Commence the
game just
over the blur
threshold

across it with your nose feather. Feel receptive and uninhibited.

2. Tell yourself what you appreciate about the image.
3. Place the photo so that it steps just over your clarity threshold into your area of blur. (Do not put the picture too far into the blur.) If you are short-sighted the picture could start out at 6 inches and later be placed at 12 inches. Or it could be that you start with the image at 2 feet and then send it to 12 feet. Far-sighted people do just the opposite.

You may scotchtape your picture to a wall, or use a chair on which to balance it. The best place to play the game is outdoors where the direct sunlight falls on to your image. The next best place to do it is indoors with light coming through a window. Or shine a strong light (150 watt spot or flood lamp) on your picture.

Relax by doing one of the basic vision improvement games. You might like to palm for five to ten minutes. Sun for a while, or do some sketching. You could combine all of these. When you feel at ease, you will be ready to transfer your relaxation and clarity into a new range.

1. With eyes open sketch a large background beyond the picture. Outline the picture itself, then sketch shapes within the picture.
2. Close your eyes and repeat the sequence. Imagine that the whole image is in the back of your head.
3. Open your eyes, stretch and yawn. Sketch the shapes in the picture once more.

Repeat steps one to three as often as you like until the images begin to change, to fluctuate. They may become clearer, larger, more colorful. Your eyes may be watering from yawning. (If you find you are trying to see, bring the picture closer so it is just within your threshold of clarity. Reestablish your relaxed attitude with one of the basic games [palming, sunning, or massage], until you know you are relaxed and receptive.)

Repeat steps one to three again.

At this point you have many options:

1. Do near-far swings with your picture. Or you might like to put another photo in your hands to provide something at close point for you to edge.

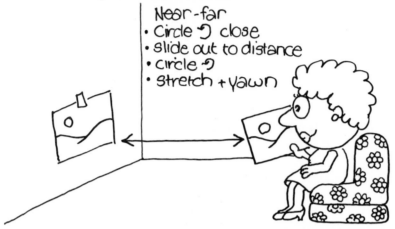

Near-far
- Circle ↺ close
- slide out to distance
- circle ↺
- stretch + yawn

2. You could play nuclear vision games as described in chapter 11. Centralize colors or elements of nature that occur in your landscape.

3. Palm and visualize yourself in the location of the photo. Imagine walking about noticing colors, fragrances and details.

You can make your own eyechart simply by cutting out black on white words from magazines and pasting them on a piece of white paper or use the charts at the back of this book. This is not the time to test or measure your vision. You are going to integrate your ability to see and relax at the same time. A formal eyechart that measures acuity isn't necessary for this although if you have one feel free to use it.

Put your eyechart and photo close together so that you are able to slide your attention and nose pencil from one to the other. Do your nose sketching on both pieces of paper.

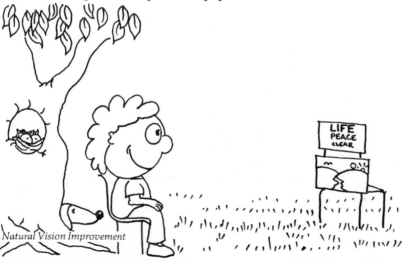

Visualize whiteness with your eyes closed. Tell yourself a white story. Then open your eyes again and scan the setting. Anything that's white — no matter how large or small, how far or near, including the white glow around eyechart letters — will announce itself to your perception. This natural way of seeing will carry you successfully past eyecharts and into the beauty of vision for as long as you like.

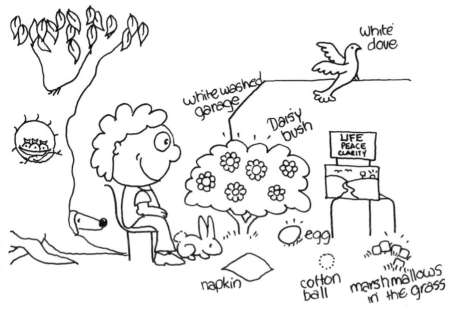

NUTRITION AND HERBS

The eyes are a window to more than the soul. The science of iridology allows us to read body conditions sometimes long before they manifest themselves as illness in the body. Vitamin deficiencies often announce their presence by visual symptoms. No question about it, what we ingest moves into and becomes the physical vehicles by which we live, enjoy and physically see. Only recently have American institutions devoted to preventing or ameliorating vision problems taken a thorough look at the effects of nutrition on both the serious eye pathologies and the startlingly prevalent myopia.

In an article bringing together various pieces of research written by Stefan Bechtel in *Prevention* of May 1982 we find out about the latest thinking. It is often 'come lately' repetition of the dietary notions that alternative doctors have been expounding for years.

We've all heard about the pilots in World War II who suffered from night blindness and were fed carrots (for vitamin A) to restore their dark perception. Recently, in Florida, an optometrist began to check for night vision as well as day vision in his clients coming in for routine eye exams. He found 26 per cent were below standard in visual ability at night and extrapolated that possibly one in four

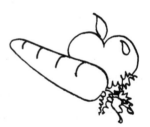

Guiding Yourself into Seeing

persons driving at night may have lowered visual ability. The Chinese have known for centuries that one looks to the liver when eye problems appear because, among other things, the liver synthesizes vitamin A.

The old-timers, Henry H. Bieler, and Alan Nittler (medical doctors who used nutrition to cure patients and were persecuted for doing so), and modern day herbalists and nutritionists look to the food we ingest to heal and revitalize the body. The plants and herbs which provide the vitamins and minerals in an organic relationship are very important. For example, students at John Hopkins Hospital demonstrated that zinc and vitamin A *together* are necessary to aid in night vision. (*Hepatology*, vol. 1, no. 4, 1981). David Knox, another doctor at Hopkins, said, 'It is extremely important for people to eat enough green and yellow vegetables to maintain normal vision.' He told *Prevention* that 'I've been studying the possibility that folic acid (vitamin B/12) or *some other unknown vitamin* from green and yellow vegetables may be essential to the maintenance of normal vision and optic nerve function.' The emphasis is the author's.

Dr Ben Lane, who is one of the consultants for Elmstrom's monograph, *Holistic Considerations for the Advancing Optometrist*, indicated that a diet full of sugar and flesh protein makes matters worse for myopes. They turn up deficient in chromium and their calcium is not utilized properly (*Documenta Ophthalmologica*, vol. 28, 1981 [1]). Chromium is necessary for the transfer of sugar in the blood stream to the tissue cells. It is absent in refined foods. A correlation between diet and eyesight keeps coming up.

My herbologist in America, Sydney Yudin, spent many years studying both Russian and Chinese herbology. He told me that every March in China the people go through a cleansing regime using herbs to rid themselves of unwelcome visitors in the intestines and to restore the vitality of the liver which is activated in the spring time. The Chinese have several herbal remedies for cataract which to them indicates an excess of phosphorus. Eyebright is used as an eye cleanser, marigold flowers for conjunctivitis. Celandine in combination with rue and cornflower, and Mi-Meng-Hua are cataract remedies.

Mi-Meng-Hua has been known in China for several thousand years. Its English name is Butterfly Bush (*Buddleia officinalis Maxim*). It clears fevers and restores clarity of vision. The conditions it is most used for are edematous and painful red eyes, bleary eyes, photophobia and blinding cataracts. It is prepared as a decoction in purified water, boiled, strained and taken internally. For more information on herbs available to doctors and herbal sources please see the Resources section at the end of this book.

People in Australia often ask me about cataract formation when I discuss the possibility of their leaving off sunglasses in this especially

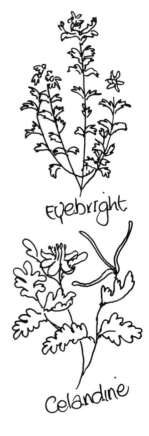

Eyebright

Celandine

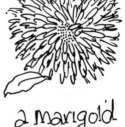

a marigold flower

brilliant landscape. They've likely heard of the survey done in Australia with 10,000 people over all parts of the country. The occurrence of cataracts was correlated with the zones of average daily sunshine. In areas of higher ultraviolet radiation there were more and earlier cataracts, especially amongst the Aborigines. The researchers made reference to the chemistry of those eyes that were developing cataracts in high sun areas. The clouding of the lens 'is inhibited by physiological levels of ascorbate (vitamin C) and glutathione (a substance that carries oxygen)' (*Lancet*, 5 Dec 1981.) In relation to skin cancer, it is Kime's book *Sunlight Can Save Your Life* which details the scientific array of data supporting ultraviolet coming into the body to *prevent* the occurrence of skin cancer. Dr Kime speculates that the ultraviolet simply hastens the tipping of the unbalanced scales when the skin is loaded with fats that prevent the cells from absorbing oxygen. Ultraviolet light is a cancer preventive when the nutritional factors of the body are in balance and when one avoids pathology-inviting circumstances such as repeated sunburns, a high fat diet, and lack of nourishing foods. Perhaps the same kind of considerations might be proffered in looking at absorption of ultraviolet, inadequate diets and the incidence of cataracts.

We've mentioned that the liver is related to eye imbalances. The kidneys may also be involved. Both these organs act as filters and cleansers for the food substances entering our mouths. After a long period of overloading the body with foods that are not assimilated or toxic in nature (caffeine, alcohol, nicotine, drugs), the liver may be overloaded. Debris starts to build up in all areas: in the bowels, the bloodstream, even the eyes. All these toxic buildups can be easily spotted in your iris by a practiced iridologist.

The liver and kidneys are given relief and an opportunity to rebuild their vital reserves by a change in diet. Sometimes guided fasting is helpful and there are herbs which will cleanse both organs.

Read all sides of the story. In a book by a trusted and experienced doctor, I read that most Americans are hypoglycemic. In a nutritional handout in an American supermarket chain their nutritionist states that hypoglycemia is an extremely rare disease. As for vegetarian versus meat-eating diets, and all the other dos and don'ts about food, let your body be your guide. Also consider that different stages of your life may call for different approaches to nutrition. When I was raising small children, I found that Bieler's diet of mainly raw or steamed vegetables, salad, fish, and chicken was perfect for me. During the past year however my body is expressing a complete disinterest in animal foods. I started to take lots of minerals, and am now happy with fresh and raw green vegetables with no cravings for sweets. This is someone talking who as a teenager fell asleep at four-o'clock every day after coming home from school — a typical hypoglycemic syndrome.

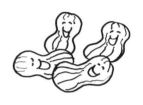

Eating is a wonderful enlivening activity. It's meant to be shared, and enjoyed, not to weigh us down or deplete our creative energy. Let's look at some ideas on eating that may please your body and brighten up your eyesight.

You are able to see the living quality of fresh, wholesome foods in their intense colors. When cooked too much or overly processed, the nutritional value and digestibility of food declines as color leaves. The brilliant green of broccoli and green beans fades to dull olive as vitamins are destroyed by long exposure to heat. When apples, cherries, or grains are ground, chopped, heated, canned, sugared and baked, they too loose their vitality. The illusion of vitality in processed foods is cast into your mind by *artificial* coloring and brilliant commercial packaging. Your body is never fooled. A persistent intake of colourless foods will eventually result in physical protests that can take the form of disease, chronic debility, and erratic emotional and mental behaviour. Consider changing your daily food habits just as you change other aspects of yourself.

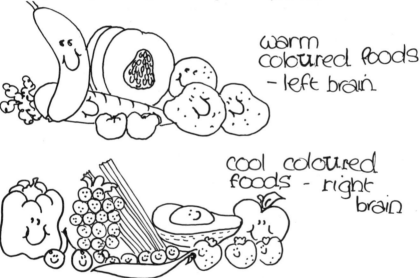

warm coloured foods - left brain

cool coloured foods - right brain

It may be helpful to consult a alternative nutritionist (one who has not been educated by vested interest groups, agribiz, or governmental agencies with subsidized foodstuffs to tout) and to peruse some of the books on nutrition listed in the Appendix.

Those people who are sugar-sensitive, hypoglycemic, or diabetic are challenged by their own sensitive natures to learn how to appropriately nourish their bodies. Many myopes with their near psychic perceptiveness appear to be as easily unbalanced by sugar as they are by unspoken feelings, gestures and environments. This imbalance makes them tense, spaced out, confused, with resulting eyestrain.

The basic guidelines are:

1. Eliminate colorless, dyed, and processed foods from your daily fare. Send the fats, sugars and salt back where they came from.
2. Eat a colorful range of food, raw or slightly cooked. Green salads and fresh vegetables could constitute the major portion of meals. Your protein may be grilled or steamed. Wholegrains are recommended. Get involved with sprouting seeds, nuts and grains. Fresh raw fruit for snacks is good.
3. If overweight, ill, specifically diseased (as in eye pathologies, cataracts, glaucoma, etc.) or subject to sluggish digestion, seek out advice and support for de-toxifying your total system. The eyes act as organs of detoxification and reflect the health of the whole body.
4. The question of vegetarian versus meat-eating diet is up to you. Your body will let you know. Research the pros and cons of each and decide for yourself. People have reported remarkable changes in their eyesight and eye health by altering their food habits.
5. Right-brain dominant people nourish themselves best with the cool-colored foods, green, blue, violet foods. Left-brain dominant folks, nourish themselves happily and readily digest the warm-colored foods. For them we generally head for the greens, yellows, oranges and reds. Notice that the starchy root vegetables are all warm colored (such as pumpkin, potatoes, beets,) and are more easily handled by the down-to-earth people than by the sensitive dreamers who thrive best on their salads, apples and berries. Green vegies are for everyone.

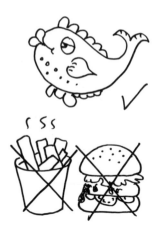

PATHOLOGIES

Glaucoma, cataract, detached retina, macular degeneration are but a few of the pathologies that appear in human eyes. These conditions are also on the rise in proportion to population. The latest figures in America show that 75 per cent of people over sixty-five have some form of cataract, a major cause of blindness. Millions of dollars are being spent in the USA on surgical procedures and lens implants with no acknowledgment of or research being done in non-surgical methods. The offical position of the American Food and Drug Administration (F.D.A.) was given to us in the November 1979 issue of the *National Health Federation Bulletin*: 'There is no approved medication for the treatment of cataracts, nor are any being investigated. Cataracts are treated in the United States solely by surgery.' There are, however, two dedicated men in California, an optometrist and an ophthalmologist, researching non-surgical nutritional treatment of cataracts that is in common use in Europe and the Orient (see Appendix for information).

The diagnosis of a pathology that may lead to blindness is frightening. It causes many people to panic and despair. Glaucoma and detached retinas are conditions that necessitate immediate diagnosis and possible treatment by an ophthalmologist. Yet once you are made aware of the best that the medical professional has to offer to save endangered eyesight, it is advisable to become informed about alternative healing — nutrition, body cleansing, homeopathy, etc. Functioning with knowledge and understanding of all the factors affecting your eyesight allows you to make decisions without fear.

Preventive means for any physical health deterioration has to do with supplying the body with appropriate nutrition, not overloading it with undigestible foods, and learning to periodically cleanse the whole system. This also involves cleansing the mind of negative thought patterns. With all cases of pathology have your medical doctor monitor the condition as you activate a natural healing program. Medical doctors are people too. Find someone who is compatible and supportive to you even if this means changing doctors or driving a bit farther.

Even if you have had surgery, or a pathology which has dimmed your sight, with the relaxation and imagery activities in this book you may be able to enjoy, enhance, and possibly maintain the vision you have now.

Chapter 17

Sharing With Others

A fair number of people have questioned in the past, 'If this Natural Vision/Bates method is so good, why isn't everyone using it?' and 'How come I've never heard of it before?'

PERSONAL RESPONSIBILITY

I juggled with a few notions in respect to the first riddle. I'd often heard the comment that eye professionals would have gone out of business if people learned to see clearly without glasses. Although this line of thinking has some merit, I feel it leads us away from a larger, more important issue. Certainly commercial interests will be defended. Yet glasses are a convenience and easy to obtain. And optometry as a career is no longer guaranteed prosperity. The marketplace is saturated with optometrists and they now have to compete with cut-rate optical outlets. It's the people, the consumers who I suspect may still not be aware of their prerogatives or potential power in the marketplace. That power and freedom of choice is often relinquished into the hands of the sellers. Today we are offered ever more facile ways of circumventing personal responsibility for our own state of being. The surgical procedure of radial keratotomy is a prime example of this. The slitting of corneas to flatten the eyes of myopes is now available at a 'reasonable' price. This pseudo-cure was commented upon in 1984 by legal attorney Bernard Freedman of Los Angeles. Mr Freedman specializes in medical malpractice cases. 'There is much controversy over and numerous medical malpractice lawsuits being filed regarding a relatively new eye surgery procedure called radial keratotomy. This is a fast and simple operation where incisions are made into the cornea to "correct" myopia. Demand for this surgery has skyrocketed althought there are questionable long-term results and numerous adverse reactions. This "quick-cure" approach to vision improvement is due to unquestioning trust being given to medical doctors by people who believe that anything a doctor does is safe and good. These myopic medical consumers become the gullible prey in a situation which is an undoubted financial windfall for a few medical practitioners.

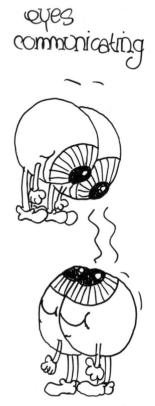

eyes communicating

Although there is no substantiated track record on the visual improvement following radial keratotomy surgery there is a record of adverse effects including glare, double vision, scarred corneas, epithelial cell loss and significant pain as well as unknown future effects on these traumatized and damaged corneas.'

Again we are brought back to the issue of personal responsibility. We are, on a grand scale, being challenged to become self-determined and self-created, starting with our own mental and physical health which includes eyesight. I am convinced that with the turning of the tide from high-tech to mature nature-harmonious ways, acknowledgment will inevitably emerge for self-healing in vision as it has done for heart disease and other cultural ailments because individuals are saying, 'this is what I want to do for and by myself'.

In mulling over the second question, 'How come I've never heard of it?', the following analysis emerged. The group of lay teachers who were teaching natural vision because of Margaret Corbett's dedication in Los Angeles, were legally proscribed from measuring, assessing, or 'proving' that their students ever had any benefit from their teaching. On the other hand, the professional, technically trained eye practitioners who were licensed to assess, measure, and determine eye performance were taught that the Bates method was ineffective, to be derided and distained. This impasse resulted in close to non-existent statistical research in alternative vision methods while millions of dollars were (and still are) being poured into cosmetic and bio-synthetic measures such as lens transplants and our new 'cure', radial keratotomy.

In addition I feel that individual optometrists and ophthalmologists have not been cognisant of the repressiveness generated through indifferent legal mechanisms fostered by professions intent on protecting their broadly defined licences.

Margaret Corbett admonished the hundreds of teachers she trained in the 1940s and 1950s never to advertise, lecture or publish articles. Some might say she was paranoid. Yet more understanding is generated by the knowledge that she was arrested (and acquitted) twice for practicing optometry without a licence. Teachers who did not heed her advice went to New York in the early 1950s. Their advertising aroused so much ire from the local optometrists that a law was passed in New York State completely proscribing the practice of the Bates method unless one had permission from a medical doctor. In 1961 the last group of Corbett-Bates teachers dissolved their association upon advice of a lawyer. The teachers scattered, lost their communication lines, and dissolved into the woodwork.

Mrs Corbett's legal battles in the 1940s was not the end of the suppression of natural vision teaching in California. In 1974 my colleague in San Francisco, Mrs Anna Kay, who'd been quietly trans-

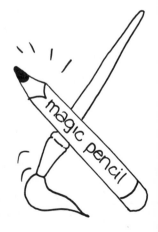

mitting Bates Method principles for several decades, was visited by two undercover agents. Subsequently she was told by the D.A.'s office that she was breaking the law on sixteen counts. The undercover investigation was generated by an article on foot reflexology that Mrs Kaye had written for a national health magazine.

In 1983, just before leaving for Australia, I received a letter from the executive officer of the Optometry Board in Sacramento. A receptionist in an optometric office had sent him one of my brochures. I must either explain to him exactly what I meant by the teaching of 'visualization' or I would face immediate investigation by the local district attorney's office. My response was to sympathize with him in that the state of California could not afford a dictionary. I mentioned that mothers teach visualization to their children when reading bedtime stories and even tennis instructors are creating champion athletes by painting certain pictures in the mind. I heard nothing further.

Both Margaret Corbett and I, following in her wake, took great care not to cross over into either the terminology or actions of eye practitioners. I had spoken on the phone with the overworked predecessor of the official gentleman just mentioned to ensure I wouldn't run afoul of the bureaucratic fortifications surrounding professional eye care. I had memorized the laws governing the practice of optometry, ophthalmology, medicine and psychology in the state of California. In my seventeen years of teaching in Los Angeles, the investigations were predictable at regular intervals. Personnel rolled over and the new blood resolutely attempted to enforce again the laws written so broadly as to threaten anyone mentioning eyes, vision, improvement, training, classes, etc. Keeping the program philosophically and practically in the area of education (which is where it thrives anyway) was the only path to follow other than making natural vision a religion. Still education in natural vision training without the use of mechanical and optical devices is simply beyond the imagination of some. That's all right. However some people think that whatever they've been exposed to is all there is. The official in Sacramento kindly advised me to obtain a licence in vision therapy and work only under *prescription of an optometrist, ophthalmologist, or licensed physician and surgeon* [emphasis his]. The medical doctors who have come into my classes as vision students came precisely because the lore I transmitted was not available through their colleagues.

The philosophy, education and methods of natural vision education lie along a completely different path from that of orthodox eye practitioners. Patient and responsible people have been and are teaching vision in their homes, schools and health centres spreading the love of vision rather than capitalizing on its vulnerability. They are practising humanness without a licence. A state of affairs I would like to see continue.

There's a third recurring query that is usually thrown at prospective students by skeptical friends or relatives. The question is 'Where's the proof? Show me some numbers. If I see real proof then I'll do it too.' You may now realize why substantiated objective proof is scarce. Only in the past two or three years have optometrists with a personal interest in alternative health begun to assess their patients who have taken some sort of Bates Method or Natural Vision course. Fortunately over the years it was always possible for me to find optometrists and finally ophthalmologists who were at least interested enough to act as objective assessors for my students. Also these practitioners had to exhibit some compatibility and graciousness during the eye exams. Otherwise students are not motivated to return to the office, either to measure progress objectively or to obtain the recommended weaker spectacles.

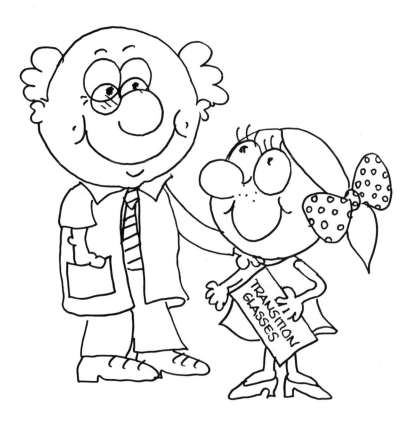

HERE'S SOME PROOF

The data in the following progress chart were gathered by optometrist H.H. Friend in 1984 in Australia. All students wearing glasses are encouraged to go to an eye practitioner to have their glasses weakened as soon as they begin a course. Mr Friend agreed to keep records showing students' progress over a fairly short period of time.

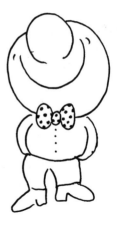

These students chose when they would return to Mr Friend's office but were advised to have their T-glasses reduced again as soon as they noticed that they were too strong. Sometimes I hear complaints that this process of reducing glasses can get expensive. With bargain opticians, optometrists willing to do partial refractions, and the use of medical benefits this rationale for not giving the eyes a chance loses all its punch.

In explanation of the chart on pages 188 & 189, we find that Miss C.B. at age twenty-seven began the vision improvement course with vision in the right eye of 6/X. The 6 signifies the distance of six meters. from the eyechart. The X means that she was unable to recognize any of the letters on the chart. The prescription (Rx) that she had been wearing to compensate for her blur was –8.50 meaning 8 and one half diopters of minus (myopic) correction in her right eye with a correction for astigmatism of two and one half diopters at the angle of 75 degrees. In her left eye she was using a lens of eight and one-quarter diopters for myopia and a correction for astigmatism of two and one quarter diopters at an angle of 165 degrees. With these glasses she was fully corrected to 6/6 metric or 20/20 in feet. Mr Friend then modified her prescription by taking out all the astigmatic correction and lowering the dioptric curvature of her myopic correction by three-quarters of a diopter in her right eye and half a diopter in her left eye. Her vision with this 'T' (Transition) Rx was then 6 over 12 which gives her adequate vision for driving. Miss C.B. then returned after four months to Mr Friend's office. With her 'T' glasses she was now reading further down the chart, showing such progress in her perception that Mr Friend was able to reduce her lenses again. This time she read the 6/12 line on the eyechart with seven diopters in the right eye and six and one-quarter diopters in the left eye. At this point she asked Mr Friend to reduce her prescription further as she was not driving a car. This requested Rx is reflected in the last column. Cases numbers two, three, four and eight denote a similar situation. These students, so pleased with their progress after years of wearing glasses, were proving their ability to see clearly with progressively weaker prescriptions.

Case #	Date	Name	Age	Unaided Vision First Visit	Rx	Vision With Glasses
1	11/83	Miss C.B.	27	R 6/X	− 8.50/− 2.50x175	6/6
				L 6/X	− 8.25/− 2.25x165	6/6
2	4/84	Mrs S.S.	34	R 6/X	− 7.00/− 0.25x135	6/6
				L 6/X	− 6.25/− 0.25x45	6/6
3	4/84	Mrs A.R.	33	R 6/48	− 2.75/− 0.50x180	6/6
				L 6/60	− 2.75/− 1.25x180	6/6
4	3/84	Mrs E.C.	33	R 6/X	− 6.50/− 1.25x150	6/6
				L 6/X	− 6.50/− 1.75x35	6/6
5	6/84	Mrs K.W.	27	R 6/38	− 2.00/− 0.25x65	6/6
				L 6/30	− 1.75	6/6
6	3/84	Mr. D.J.A.	31	R 6/48	− 3.00/− 0.25x60	6/6
				L 6/30	− 3.25/− 0.75x75	6/6
7	3/84	Miss J.B.	27	R 6/75	− 0.25/− 1.50x40	6/6
				L 6/84	− 1.75/− 2.50x130	6/6
8	3/84	Miss J.B.	29	R 6/X	− 4.25/− 3.25x165	6/6
				L 6/X	− 4.75/− 1.75x15	6/6
9	2/	Mrs J.Mc.		R 6/75	Plano	6/75
				L 6/75	+ 0.75/− 0.50x135 Add + 0.75	6/75

Modified Rx for 'T' Glasses	Vision With 'T' Rx	Returned After	Vision With 'T' Rx	Modified Rx	Vision With new 'T' Rx	Given
−7.75	6/12		6/7	−7.00	6/12	−6.75
		4 months				
−7.75	6/12		6/9.5	−6.25	6/12	−6.00
−6.00	6/12			−5.75	6/12	−5.00
		3 month				
−5.50	6/12			−4.75	6/12	−3.50
−2.25	6/12			−1.50	6/12	−1.00
		1 week				
−2.50	6/12			−2.00	6/12	−1.50
−6.25	6/12		6/6	−5.75	6/12	−3.00
		2 months				
−6.25	6/12		6/7.5	−5.75	6/12	−3.00
−1.25	6/12		6/95	−1.00	6/12	
		4 months				
−0.75	6/12		6/12	−0.50	6/12	
−2.00	6/12			−1.75	6/12	
		3 weeks				
−2.25	6/12			−1.75	6/12	
−0.25	6/12			Plano	6/9.5	
		1 month				
−1.50 −1.25x130	6/12			−1.00	6/12	
−4.25 −1.50x165	6/12		6/12	−4.25	6/12	−3.75
		3 months				
−4.75 −0.50x150	6/12		6/12	−4.00	6/12	−3.75
no glasses far	6/75		6/6	Reads without glasses far and near		
		1 month				
or near	6/75		6/6			

Case no.	Original Rx	Present Rx	Vision BE	Vision w/o Rx	Estimated % improvement objectively measured.
1	− 3.75/+ 1.00x100 − 3.25/+ 1.00x 95	− 1.50 − 1.50	20/15	Day 20/25 Night 20/50	54%
2	− 2.25 − 2.25	− 1.00 − 1.00	20/20	Day 20/40 Night 20/50	56% 56%
3	− 4.25/+ 1.75x120 − 3.25/+ 0.75x4	− 1.75 − 1.50	20/20	Day 20/40 Night 20/70	50%
4	− 7.75/+ 1.50x10 − 7.25/+ 1.25x0	− 4.50 − 4.00	20/25		30%
5	− 5.00/+ 2.00x95 − 3.50/+ 1.75x90	− 2.50 − 1.00	20/25	Day 20/25 Night 20/50	50%
6	− 3.25/+ 0.50x0 − 3.50/+ 1.50x95	− 1.00 − 1.00	20/25		65%
7	− 8.00/+ 0.75x80 − 7.75/+ 0.50x90	− 4.00 − 4.00	20/30		45%
9	− 3.25/+ 0.50x150 − 2.25	− 2.00 − 1.25	20/20	Day 20/40 Night 20/80	40%
10	− 8.75/+ 2.25x90 − 7.00/+ 2.25x95	− 7.00 = + 0.75x90 − 6.00 = + 0.75x90	20/25		15%
11	− 2.50/+ 0.75x83 − 3.00	− 0.75 − 1.50	20/20		60%
12	− 3.00/+ 0.56x175 − 3.50/+ 0.75x35	− 1.50 − 1.50	20/20	w/o correction 20/40	50%
13	− 3.25/+ 0.75x177 − 4.00/+ 1.00x176	− 2.50 − 2.50	20/15	w/o correction 20/70	30%
14	+ 4.00 + 3.25	+ 1.75 + 1.75	20/20 near point	went back to + 2.75 BE 20/20	30%
15	− 6.50 − 9.00 (20/30)	− 5.50 − 7.50	20/30		30%
16	− 9.00/+ 0.50x05 − 4.75/+ 0.75x05	− 6.00 − 3.00	20/50		30%
17	plano/+ 3.25x140 plano/+ 2.50x44	+ 1.50x175 + 1.50x55	20/20	can see 20/20 w/o correction	50% +
18	+ 3.00 reading + 2.25/+ 0.75x96	+ 1.75 + 0.75 + + 1.75x70	20/20		40%

The data on the left page was established by ophthalmologist J. Soorani in Los Angeles in 1980-84. The case numbers represent students who attended an eight to twelve week class series taught by me or by one of my certified teachers.

The above data were gathered on these case people over time periods ranging from two to three weeks for cases 9, 10, and 13, to one to three years. Most of these students would have taken an eight to ten week course and then continued on their own. We do not know what would have happened if these people had continued to take courses, or had been given refresher weekends. Cases number 5, 13, and 15, in spite of their objectively demonstrated improvements, chose for unknown reasons to return to their original prescriptions. A future charting of natural vision improvement students' progress might well include the hours spent in classes and autobiographical stories. The objectively measured data given above clearly demonstrates that 'irreversible' myopia is amenable to improvement.

In 1977, Coralie La Salle conducted a study of twelve myopic students attending vision classes and private lessons which I taught. Her thesis, titled 'Some Psychophysiological Influences in Myopia', included the following measurements which were made by a licensed optometrist in the Los Angeles area. Coralie was awarded a master's degree from UCLA for this study. She became a certified teacher and works in Los Angeles.

Subject	Beginning Acuity		Ending Acuity		Months in Training
M1	R20/400	L20/400	R20/400	L20/300	15
F1	20/600	20/400	20/500	20/400	3
F2	20/300	20/80	20/70	20/60	7
F3	20/800	20/800	20/500	20/500	6
M2	20/400	20/200	20/300	20/100	4
F4	20/400	20/400	2/200	20/200	10
F5	20/250	20/250	20/200	20/200	6
F6	20/400	20/400	20/200	20/200	3
F7	20/400	20/400	20/300	20/300	3
F8	20/600	20/600	20/600	20/600	12
F9	20/600	20/600	20/600	20/600	11
F10	20/800	20/800	20/60	20/60	1½*

The starred line is the data for Barbara Hughes who became the first certified teacher in Natural Vision Improvement. She resided at my home in California for her training and went on to write a book called *Twelve Weeks to Better Vision*.

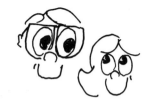

PERSONAL STORIES

The following are just a few of the many letters vision students have sent.

13 August 1981

Dear Janet:

After attending your vision training class for three months I wanted to write and tell you my experience. First of all, I think you are doing something important and valuable and I want to acknowledge your perseverance in the face of not a lot of agreement in the medical community. I enjoyed the classes, learned a lot and have a totally different perspective on my aging vision. I have dispensed with my reading and sun glasses and am doing many of your exercises as often as I remember to do them. Since they are simple and enjoyable I think I can keep up the program indefinitely. I noted that all my classmates were progressing and enjoying the program as much as I was.

As I mentioned I hope someday to incorporate a similar vision training program in the preventive medicine-health enhancement program of which I am currently medical director. The attitudes about vision and glasses which you advocate fit perfectly with our own approach to patient education and enlightenment in the area of optimal health.

Thank you for the enormous contribution you have made to my own, and to your other students' understanding of vision and the human potential.

Cleaves M. Bennett, M.D
Medical Director
Innerhealth Program
Los Angeles, California, USA

5 May 1981

Dear Janet:

I had been wearing glasses for six years and I dreaded every moment of it. I started out needing reading glasses, then my distance vision became impaired and I found myself in bifocals. Being a physically active person, glasses were definitely a handicap. I felt I was doomed to wear glasses forever.

About five months ago I found I was in need of a stronger prescription as my eyes were growing weaker. My wife had heard of your natural vision improvement classes and urged me to look into your class. As you already know, I did just that. In just a few short months my vision has returned to normal.

Thanks to you and your natural vision class I have thrown my glasses away. Being in the field of Business Management and Accounting it's such a joy to work without glasses. Just last month I renewed my driver's licence without glasses. I recommend you to everyone I meet wearing glasses.

*Again, thank you so much for helping me improve my sight
the natural way.*
A.L. Dwyer
Pasadena, California, USA

1982

Dear Janet:
*As a holistic health educator, I experienced an extraordinary
burst of energy through my eyes in your vital eyes class. My glasses
are now gathering dust in my desk.*
Elly Wagner, B.A.
Los Angeles, California, USA

5 July 1984

Dear Janet:
*Hello and a big hug to you. I loved your workshops. I have
been having more exciting dreams and my eyesight has also improv-
ed dramatically. My initial statistics back in March of 1984 were:*
R: −4.25 − 3.25×165 L: −4.75−1.75×15
My modified prescription:
R: −4.25 − 1.50×165 L: −4.75−0.50×15
And improvement on 17 June 1984 another modified prescription:
R: −3.75   L: −3.75
Needless to say, I was very excited. Lots of love, happy dreaming,
Judy Barclay
Melbourne, Victoria, Australia

November 1984

Dear Janet:
*Unfortunately I was under a lot of stress during my pregnancy
with Paul. I was tired and couldn't sleep. When he was born he
seemed in perfect health. His eyes appeared perfectly straight. But
at the age of six weeks both eyes turned in almost to the point where
the pupils were disappearing. His eyes were doing this together or
alternately. At two months we become very concerned. My husband, having had similiar problems in his babyhood, was operated
on at seven years of age, suffered shortsightedness, wears glasses,
and had no fusion. We got a referral to an eye specialist who wanted
to operate on both eyes within the next two weeks. Paul was three
months old. I was most distressed and became very anxious knowing about the failure and damage of eye operations . . . I believed*

there must be some other way. My sister, Mary, had glasses and had been to one of your workshops. She gave me your phone number. I was pleased to meet you and learn all the games that you have taught us to help Paul. I now feel I'm an important vision teacher to Paul. But with the pressure from friends and relations, I took Paul once again to the eye and ear hospital. The eye specialist had never heard of eye exercises and his only answer was to operate. He admitted that he couldn't guarantee the delicate operation would be successful and it might have do be done more than once. I thought 'forget it'. In this time I had also visited another eye specialist. I found him a most considerate and patient man. Paul was four months old. He took time and explained to me about the muscles pulling too tightly. And he felt that there was no way Paul needed to be operated on. Paul is now 16 months old and is improving. I am sure this is because we are tuned in to what is happening with his vision. We play with him what we have learned from you (whom we still see on occasion). I still take him for periodic checks to see if his sight is developing in both eyes. As long as Paul keeps on improving the doctor will not interfere in any way. I feel I've been a caring and responsible parent and that I am doing as much as possible for Paul as I'm able. His father took the adult course to help Paul and himself. Paul won't go through his Dad's experience because he is off to a better start.

Anne McDougal
Melbourne, Victoria, Australia

November 1984

Dear Janet:

This is something I wrote which I give to people who ask, 'How did you hear about Janet?'

Rushing home for lunch one day in 1981 I switched on the TV. Mike Walsh was in the centre of an interview with a woman advocating Natural Vision — no spectacles. I WAS INTERESTED, as I'd found reading glasses my largest frustration about getting old. Over ten years ago I'd found outlines getting fuzzy and had to resort to reading glasses. Reading became a hassle but that was minor in comparison with so many other activities that had been easy or a pleasure. I couldn't read the dials on the kitchen stove or my recipes, so glasses in the kitchen were essential and then they got fogged up in the steam. Also numbers on the telephone; letters on the typewriter; prices in the shops and the time by my watch. All demanded a search for glasses. Finally expensive multi-focal lenses were the answer but I soon found myself living in these. Certainly at work they were never off. But what of pleasures? Reading in bed had lost its attraction as the pillow pushed the glasses out of focus. Handcraft by the TV was also out, as constant focusing was irritating. Music was a nightmare. And lastly vanity. No hair-do could look attractive around my small face as the glasses altered the contour and pushed all the hair up and out at the ears. Earrings too, had always looked good but they became no nos because earrings, gold chain and glasses were so much that I felt like a gypsy with all the dangles and baubles. So ... bliss, the thought of dispensing with the irritation that I had been led to believe inevitable in old age, was a delight. I wrote to the TV station and found out the woman was Janet Goodrich. Unfortunately, at that time she was on tour and unavailable for teaching. In September 1983 she returned to lecture and hopefully set up schools on her work here in Australia. I attended her vision workshop in Melbourne.

As we arrived, we sat in a large circle in the loungeroom; she interviewed us separately and told us all to put our glasses away. It was an ordeal and I inwardly scoffed at the thought that I would never need them again. But I haven't ... from that moment to this.

So we began ... first yawning. Yawn. Yawn. And more yawning, as she stressed relaxation of the neck and face muscles; and as our eyes teared and noses ran, we took deep breaths, great yawns and loud noises as we exhaled. Then she began a series of psychological tests to make sure that both sides of the brain were switched on. This, with lecturing, explanations and physical exercises for 'switching on' the both sides of the brain, took up all the first day. At this stage I knew very little about Dr Bates, who in the 1920s had first conceived these ideas. I drove home after that first night feeling let down, nothing had been done about eyes, about seeing. I'd 'done my dough' I thought. I had a tremendous headache ... so much for all the relaxation! So I did nothing that night and went to bed disillusioned thinking that the whole thing was a hoax. But I'd paid my money so I may well see what happened the next day.

On the Sunday it was a perfect spring day in Melbourne so Janet took us into the garden in the sunlight. I had always hated the sun, its heat and glare causing me distress and I said so as I headed for the shade. This, she said was a mistake — I must change my thinking and learn to 'love the sun' as the source of all light for human vision. So we began to talk as we sat in the sunshine. We did more yawning, breathing, relaxing and then began to learn the new concepts for reading, by seeing the white at the back of the black letters and allowing the black letters to jump out at us. This new concept (continues to take practice) combined with other activities such as palming, edging, sunning, near and far imaginings, etc, were utterly new to us all. BUT, by noon I read from a small vision card, a paragraph where the print was so small I'd not even known it was there at the beginning of the morning. To begin I'd found the top line of large letters a blur, but by noon I could read the entire card.

This 'flash' of what was possible was, to me, so remarkable as to be miraculous. I came home on the plane, and for the first time was able to read the seat number on my boarding pass. I did my knitting in the plane and I could see the stitches. I arrived home in such a state of jubilant excitement I was as a new-born Christian must have felt in the early days of Christianity. Of course, as with the early Christians we all have ups and downs, but the downs are minor, when I'm tired or in a poor light, and I have never again worn glasses.

My first day at work was traumatic 'How would I manage?' I kept asking myself. I saw the rows of pink and yellow borrowing cards as a blur, but I remembered the principle of the reading lesson and I practised them until gradually the blurs distinguished themselves as names, and I was content. So it was with everything I did — my mail, my typewriter, the books in the library. The tiny print of an index, a map, a telephone book, I am not yet able to read clearly, but I have the pin spot specs that Janet gave us and I use these as my panic glasses. They are merely black plastic with tiny holes in them, no glass at all, but they enable me to see clearly, for that one small instant and are never worn continually. But it is so long now since I've needed them that they are gathering dust in the bottom of my handbag.

So it is that I recommend this wonderful way of seeing. Janet came to Hobart in January 1984 and ran a similar weekend in my home here. She also gave advice, interviews, a public lecture to 250 people. It was a full and rewarding time and showed me more than ever how vital this work is to such a variety of people. The method works for all, no matter what the problem, as it is all based on relaxation and the natural use of the eye, the mind and the body. When all these are in harmony, clear vision results. This is the delight also, that anyone can see clearer, get brighter colours and have no eyestrain.

Since finding this for myself I've read more books and vision magazines and see just how many people have proven its success. I now feel almost as I always did. I have confidence in my eyes and no need to seek glasses. I feel relaxed and happy no matter how much reading, etc I do. I've done very little 'special' work, but in a rushed life, I put the practice into every day use. I hope I may still do more to improve the really close-up work and detail as I'm sure is possible. I still want to do a lot of fine embroidery with counting threads in the material and to do this eyesight must be perfect. When I can again do that I'll have reached my goal — for the present I'm so happy with all other activities that I'm letting it wait for that every elusive 'more time'.

Judy Barber
Hobart, Tasmania, Australia

The following progress reports were written by students in the fifth week of an eight week public course. They were meeting once a week for two hours with certified natural vision teachers Doreen Cott and Keith Millar.

22 November 1984

Dear Keith:

Last Saturday, I graced the shores of Half Moon Bay and did heaps of sunning exercises. To my total surprise I saw the face of my friend clearly — every single line. I wept from sheer frustration, he wept for joy!

Absolutely fantastic course — my job is fairly high stress — not conducive to vision improvement, but you've taught me how to relax, pity it wasn't twenty years ago.

I feel less like a 'blind' person and I don't give a stuff if I can't see peoples' faces yet — I will, even if I don't I feel much more confident about walking into a room and not seeing much.

Many, many, many thanks — you've not only influenced me but all the people I will ever meet.

Barbara Bereznicki
Melbourne, Victoria, Australia

22 November 1984

In 5 weeks, I have learned to relax, see much better, still use glasses to read, but not for short periods anymore. I notice variations in my vision more than before. There is a definite improvement of my general vision.

Manfred J. Chlupac
Melbourne, Victoria, Australia

22 November 1984

After five weeks training, I am more aware of holding my breath when I concentrate and how tense I have been. The neck exercises and breathing and yawning are greatly relaxing. Palming is just terrific and I can see so clearly for a few minutes afterwards — so relaxing I feel terrific.

I am more aware of what I can see now and only wear glasses when I feel I have to. When I do wear my glasses, I am now aware of what I can't see through them. I also realize that before I was rarely out in the sun at all without glasses, now I am a lot.

I noticed after sewing recently my eyes are not so tired as before I started this course.

Mary King
Melbourne, Victoria, Australia

22 November 1984

After five weeks training, I can do bookwork without my glasses for awhile, sometimes the whole morning, but sometimes only a short time.

Only very occasionally have I used my stronger glasses. I can sometimes write without my glasses and once I wrote a seven page letter without them. I used to wear sunglasses nearly all of the time while driving, now I can very often go without them, but still need them when driving into the sun.

Outside I am able to see better, doing bookwork. Unfortunately it is often too cold, too hot or I have too many things to take out. I have some trouble with palming. I find it very difficult to sit there any longer than a few minutes knowing I have so much to do. I do most exercises two or three times a day.

Elly Ranten
Melbourne, Victoria, Australia

22 November 1984

I can now write without glasses. I am now aware of the amounts of tension and strain from old visual habits and its effect on vision. I get lots of energy from the 'switching on' movements.

Barbara Lancaster (5th class)
Melbourne, Victoria, Australia

22 November 1984

I am now in the fifth week of class. It seems to be easier to see things more clearly (I used to stare a lot, having my mind on something else).

Playing the piano has become less tiring. I had problems with reading the music and looking down on the keys in rapid speed. The notes were not blurred, but they sort of floated into each other, my eyes didn't move fast enough. I notice that I am also able to concentrate better.

I had an interesting dream: I was alone in a strange unlighted room and noticed that there actually was light around myself, moving with me as I moved through the room.

Colors seem to be brighter too. Did some palming last night: it was absolutely black and I felt drawn into a void, floating, very relaxing and pleasant.

Gudour Markowsky
Melbourne, Victoria, Australia

22 November 1984

Now I notice how my vision fluctuates. When things are blurry, I am prompted to blink and edge and do near-far swings to create clarity. My eyes feel as if they have more energy and they don't get so tired when I'm reading or working. I am also driving with more confidence.

Rosalind Harding (5th class)
Melbourne, Victoria, Australia

22 November 1984

My dreams are now easier to remember and more frequent. I am noticing fine detail more such as the veins on a flower petal, and I was a presbyope.

My thinking process has become clearer and I'm able to come up with alternatives to problems.

I am able to visualize better when I'm reading which leads to better understanding. Colors are sharper and brighter. Already I am in weaker glasses.

M. Lanassa (5th class)
Melbourne, Victoria, Australia

22 November 1984

Dear Doreen

I participated in a Weekend Vision Workshop and have since noticed wonderful improvements. The world is more colorful. Night driving is easier. I no longer experience glare from headlights. My peripheral vision has switched-on. Reading is easier because the black is blacker. I have been happier and more alert and relaxed and my appreciation of art is developing. I'm in my second pair of weaker glasses. My astigmatism correction has gone from −2 to −1 which is 50% improvement! The vision workshop that I did was one of the best things I've ever done in my life.

Joe Micallif
Melbourne, Victoria, Australia

A seven year old natural vision student shares with us:

'I'm seven years old and in the second grade. Last year the nurse said I had to wear glasses so I got some. I don't like them much cause they're always sliding around and I have to take care of them. But they helped me see some stuff clearer. Now my mom and dad are starting to do other things with me. After supper, we all sit at the table for a while and cover our eyes. We tell funny stories and talk about trips we've been on. Then we massage on the bones around our eyes. We move our legs and arms like we're crawling. Then I go outside, and play with my big red ball against the wall of my house. In the morning before I go to school, my dad and I lean up against his car and do some sunning. My folks sent a note to my teacher telling her about what we're doing — teaching my eyes and body to relax so I can see better without glasses. It's nice. I get my shoulders massaged and do other fun things like dancing around and yawning a lot. At first I thought all this stuff was really silly. I was into watching TV and reading comics more. I still do that but I do other things too. Yah, no more soda pop and candy except for special times. My vision is getting better. The eye doctor was happy when we went. Oh yes, I forgot to tell you. When I learn about something new in school, I always close my eyes for a bit and draw it with my nose. Yesterday I drew whales and now I remember all about them.

A MESSAGE FROM A NATURAL VISION TEACHER

The great thing about being a teacher of vision is that your own vision is getting better all the time and I'm able to say this even though I've never worn glasses myself.

It is rewarding to see people change and reveal their true natures. I just listen to what my students tell me about their experiences with their vision, seeing things differently than they have in years. It's exciting when people learn to get more pleasure from their vision and it's also interesting to hear how activation of the right hemisphere manifests in other areas of their lives such as creativity, ability to recall dreams, relaxation, more energy, and more happiness in general.

Glasses inhibit the natural movement and expressions of the body as much as they do the movement of the eyes. Think about it the next time you have your glasses on and you feel an urge to bend over or upside down or shake your head energetically. Do you stifle the feeling or hold back from moving wholeheartedly rather than upset the delicate balance of the foreign object on your nose? Or are you determined enough to take them off and have a go at some wild movement letting yourself go and freeing up your whole body and then put the glasses on only to walk stiffly and sedately out of the room until the next time you are bold enough to do it again? Wearing glasses is as much a straight jacket for the body as for the eyes. Adults and children alike come to me with restricted movement of the head and neck which leads to energy blockages in the cervical spine, and furthering the deterioration of the eyes. This situation results from the purely physical demands of keeping glasses on the face. I have noticed that even laughter is restricted with glasses on. People refrain from throwing their heads back and enjoying a good belly laugh for fear of having their glasses fly off and break. Since body movement facilitates eye movements, I emphasize total body/dance movements integrated with eye movements, (swinging and blinking) in order to free up the entire visual system. You must break both the stare of the body as well as the eyes. When I worked with a particular little girl named Rebecca (aged seven), I became aware of how much she loved to move her body. Rebecca was myopic When she would arrive for her lesson, having just left school, tension was blatantly noticable throughout her body. She would walk in quietly and carefully, sit down shyly and express minimal movement. Coming from the school environment, kids will be particularly tight, holding their breath so that yawning takes a long time to come through. They are switched-off and sluggish. Their personalities and energy levels would radically change by the end of the lesson. Rebecca moved freely, laughed easily and was happily loosened up when she left, looking forward to the next lesson. The best approach for her was to get her body moving, which in turn freed up her breathing and her eyes.

Doreen Cott

TEACHER TRAINING

Certified instructors have been trained in Natural Vision Improvement in courses given around the world. The advantages of having a teacher comes from the personal contact with someone who has gained the experience and the knowledge to support, in a caring way, the vision of others. It is not necessary that you wear glasses or that your vision is 20/20 to become a candidate for the instructor's course. If you are interested in further details, please complete the coupon below in legible print and send it along with a self addressed stamped envelope to

Janet Goodrich, Ph.D.
Natural Vision Improvement,

Celestial Arts
900 Modoc Street
Berkeley
California 94707
U.S.A.

All improvements in vision are significant, as well as advances in attitude, eye comfort and functioning. If you have used this program to your advantage and pleasure please write to me about it, including any optometric records if convenient. Your story will be added to the growing trove of empirical statements about peoples' ability to heal their own sight.

Janet Goodrich, Ph.D.
Natural Vision Improvement
Celestial Arts
900 Modoc Street
Berkeley
California 94707
U.S.A.

I am interested in:
☐ contacting a certified teacher
☐ instructors' training
☐ lectures
☐ workshops, classes
    (in Australia, N.Z., Europe, the U.S.)

☐ I would like to sponsor a workshop in my area.

NAME _____
ADDRESS _____
CITY & STATE _____
COUNTRY _____ POSTCODE _____
DATE _____

Biographies

Dr William Bates was born in New Jersey in 1860. He specialized in ophthalmology and was drawn to developing his techniques of vision improvement based on relaxation of muscles and visualization when he became dissatisfied with the use of artificial lenses to correct refractive error. In his research, Bates proved that the normal fixation of the eye is central, but never stationary.

Dr Bates was a quiet modest man, a serious student of literature and astronomy, a spontaneous and fond father. He died in 1931, a recognized eminent ophthalmologist, but his major work on visual theory was rejected by conventional medicine.

Wilhelm Reich, M.D. was a psychiatrist and scientist who trained with Sigmund Freud in Vienna. Reich broke away from the mainstream of verbal psychoanalysis to develop and substantiate his own theories that mental and emotional aberrations become locked into body musculature. His ideas reverberate today through the areas of natural childbirth, alternative schooling, life positive sexuality, body and breathing therapies, bioenergetics, gestalt, psychosomatic medicine, even weather control and UFOs. Reich backed up his comprehensive approach to mental and social illness by careful scientific studies. Many of these were burned in the Long Island incinerator after he had been sentenced to two years imprisonment for refusing to submit to a court order arbitrating the value of his work. He died in federal prison in the USA in 1957.

Margaret Darst Corbett was born in Boston, 1890, became a vision instructor after her husband's long-term poor vision and health were restored with the aid of the Bates method. Corbett then devoted her life to setting up a school to train teachers with many branches in the USA and other countries. She endured and won legal battles for practicing optometry without a licence. She taught quietly until her death at 71, having achieved the successful training of many teachers in her method.

Appendix

REFERENCES

Arguelles, Jose and Miriam *Mandala*. Berkeley and London: Shambala, 1972.

Barefoot Doctor's Manual, *A Guide to Traditional Chinese and Modern Medicine*. Washington, D.C.: United States Government Printing Office. **A sourcebook for Chinese Herbology.**

Bates, William H. *Better Eyesight Without Glasses*.

Bieler, Henry *Food Is Your Best Medicine*.

Buzan, Tony *Use Both Sides Of Your Brain*. New York: E.P. Dutton, 1974.

Caplan, Frank *The First Twelve Months of Life*. New York: Bantam.

Caplan, Theresa and Frank *The Second Twelve Months of Life, The Early Childhood Years: The 2- to 6-Year-Old*. New York: Bantam, 1983.

Clark, Linda *Color Therapy*. Old Greenwich, Connecticut: Devin-Adair, 1975.

Corbett, Margaret D. *Help Yourself To Better Sight*. North Hollywood, California: Wilshire Books. **Explanation of the Bates Method and simple techniques.**

Delacato, Carl H. *The Treatment and Prevention of Reading Problems*. Springfield III: Charles C. Thomas Co., 1959.

Dennison, Paul *Switching On*. Glendale, California: Edu-Kinesthetics, Inc. 1981. **This book is written for lay people and teachers.**

Diamond, John *Your Body Doesn't Lie*. New York: Warner.

Drury, Neville ed. *Bodyworks*.

Dufty, William *Sugar Blues*. New York: Warner, 1975.

Duke-Elder, Sir Steward *Ophthalmic Optics and Refraction*. London: Henry Kimpton, 1970.

Edwards, Betty *Drawing On The Right Side Of The Brain*, **A course in enhancing creativity and artistic confidence.** Los Angeles: Tarcher, Inc. 1979.

Ekman, Paul, and Friesen, Wallace *Unmasking The Face*. New Jersey: Prentice-Hall, 1975.

Elmstrom, George *Holistic Consideration For The Advancing Optometrist*. Chicago III, The Professional Press, Monograph Series 8201, 1983. **Written for optometrists, this monograph suggests a good look be taken at the effects of nutrition on eyesight.**

Ferguson Marilyn, ed. *The Brain Mind Bulletin*, Volume 7, Number 17, 25 Oct 1982.

Gelwey, Timothy *The Inner Game of Tennis and the Inner Game of Golf.*

Gesell, Arnold, Ilg, Francis L., and Bullis G.E. *Vision: Its Development in Infant and Child*. New York: Hefner, 1949, reprinted 1967.

Gottlieb, Raymond L. Neuropsychology Of Myopia. *J. Optom. Vis. Devel.* 13(1); 3-27, 1982.

Hall, Dorothy *Iridology. Personality and Health Analysis Through The Iris.* Melbourne: Nelson, 1980.

Harmon, Darrell Boyd *Restrained Performance As A Contributing Cause of Visual Problems*. OEP Research Reports.

_____ 'The Coordinated Classroom' in *The Nation's Schools,* March 1950.

Harrison, John *Love Your Disease. It's Keeping You Healthy*. Sydney: Angus & Robertson Publishers, 1984.

Henderson, Hazel *Alternative Futures.* New York: Berkeley Windhover Books, 1978

Horn, Ross *The Health Revolution* Sydney, 1981.

Hughes, Barbara *Twelve Weeks To Better Vision*. New York: Pinnacle, 1981. **Barbara gives her personal story of improving myopia in addition to basic activities and discussion of technical aspects underlying impaired vision.**

Huxley, Aldous *The Art Of Seeing*. Seattle: Montana Books, 1975. **Aldous Huxley, out of his gratitude to Margaret Corbett and his love of the concepts of the Bates method, wrote this book which was first published in 1942.**

Jones, Barry *Sleepers, Wake, Technology and the Future of Work.* Melbourne: OWP, 1982.

Kelley, Charles R. 'Psychological Factors In Myopia'. *J. Am. Optom. Assoc.*, 33(6): 833-837, 1967.

Kavner, Richard S. L.D., and Dusky, Lorraine *Total Vision*. New York: A & W Visual Library. 1978.

Kime, Zane, M.D., M.S. *Sunlight Could Save Your Life*. Penryn, California: World Health Publication. **Highly recommended book, easy to read, full of information and references for lay people and professionals.**

Li-Shih-Chen *Chinese Herbal Medicine*. Translated by F. Porter Smith, M.D., and G.A. Stuart, M.D., San Francisco: Georgetown Press, 1973.

Leboyer, F. *Birth Without Violence*. London: Wildwood House, 1975.

Lowen, Alexander *The Betrayal of the Body*. London: Collier Macmillan, 1967.

Mendelsohn, Robert, *Confessions Of A Medical Heretic*. New York: Warner.

Lüscher, Max, and Scott, Ian. *The Lüscher Color Test*. New York: Random House 1969.

Ott, John *Health & Light*. Old Greenwich, Connecticut: Devin-Adair, 1973.

_____ *Light, Radiation, And You*. Old Greenwich, Connecticut: Devin-Adair.

Pentecost, Marlene *Cooking for Your Life*. Sydney: Reed, 1982.

Reich, Wilhelm *Selected Writings, An Introduction to Orgonomy*. New York: Farrar, Straus and Giroux. 1951-1973. **Particularly 'The Expressive Language of the Living'.**

_____ *Character Analysis*. New York: Farrer, Straus, and Giroux, 1972.

Reubin, David M.D. *Everything You Always Wanted to Know About Nutrition*. Boston: G.K. Hall & Co., 1979.

Samuels, Mike, and Samuels, Nancy *Seeing With the Mind's Eye*. New York: Random House, 1975.

Scholl, Lisette *Visionetics*. New York: Doubleday, 1978. **A combination of Corbet-Bates methods, Neo-Reichian techniques, yoga and journal keeping.**

Shorr, Joseph D. *Go See The Movie in Your Head*. New York: Popular Library, 1977.

Stafford, Julie *Taste of Life*. Melbourne: Greenhouse, 1983.

Tobe, John *Cataract Glaucoma and Other Eye Disorders*. St. Catharines, Ontario, 1973. **Thorough discussion of nutrition as it relates to eye diseases.**

Walther, David S. *Applied Kinesiology*, Vol 1 Basic Procedures and Muscle Testing. Pueblo, Colorado: Systems DC 1981. **This book is an excellent textbook for professionals interested in the precision use of muscle testing to restore health. Written mainly for chiropractors it is also of use to dentists, optometrists, psychologists and medical doctors.**

Yarbus, Alfred L. *Eye Movements and Vision*. New York; Plenum Press, 1967.

OTHER RESOURCES

Herbs: Health practitioners anywhere in the world upon request will receive a catalogue of herbal formulas from Sidney Yudin, Dean of the College of Oriental Medicine and Professor of Herbology at Union University, Los Angeles, by writing to: Little Herb Company, 515 West Allen Ave 3, San Dimas, California 91773

Health Rights Organizations: The following group publishes regular bulletins on alternative health care and governmental legislation affecting public access to alternate methods of healing: National Health Federation, 212 W. Foothill Blvd. Monrovia, California, 91016.

Optometric Visual Training: Information can be obtained from Optometric Extension Program Foundation Inc, Duncan, Oklahoma 73533, USA.

Brain balancing and total health for lay people. Classes and seminars are available through the Touch for Health Foundation, 1174 N. Lake Ave. Pasadena, California, 91104
There is also a network of people across the country using cross-crawl and emotional balancing. Contact Educational Kinesthetics: P.O. Box 5002, Glendale, California, 91201.
Also, Three In One Concepts, 3210 West Burbank Blvd. Suite A, Burbank, California, 91505
For a list of publications by John Diamond, M.D. on the effects of environment, language, breathing, music on creativity, send to The Institute for Life Enhancement and Creativity. Post Office Drawer 37, Valley Cottage, New York, N.Y. 10989

Eyepatches: Eyepatches may be ordered by the dozen from Snugfit Eye Patch Company, P.O. Box 264, Yucaipa, California, 92399

Pinhole Spectacles: Write to Diana Deimel, 32880 Olive Avenue, Dept. G., Winchester, California 92396, USA for current price and availability.

Glossary

ACCOMMODATION: The ability of the visual system to see clearly in the distance and up close.

ALTERNATIVE MEDICINE A way of thinking about disease that recognizes the connection between body and mind. Methods for alleviating disease and preventing illness by considering the person as a whole rather than treating symptoms. Includes lifestyle changes such as diet, thinking patterns, exercise, the use of herbs, touch, chiropractic, etc.

AMBLYOPIA (LAZY EYE) reduced vision uncorrectable by glasses. It occurs when the brain 'switches off' the messages coming from an eye.

ARMORING The word coined by Wilhelm Reich to describe the chronic tightness of body muscles resulting from repression of emotional feelings. This armoring may manifest itself in eye muscles as well as in other parts of the body.

ASTIGMATISM The blurring of lines at a particular angle. This condition comes and goes and is possibly caused by stressful posture, physical distortions, and emotional factors. Metaphorically, the inability to accept.

AUTONOMIC NERVOUS SYSTEM That part of our nervous system that functions automatically and is in charge of maintaining a stable internal environment.

BATES METHOD A way of relaxing and mobilizing the whole visual system devised by American ophthalmologist William H. Bates. This method emphasized the connection between the body and mind and gave individuals a way to improve their sight without depending on glasses or professionals.

BEHAVIORAL OPTOMETRY A specialized branch of optometry which recognizes the influence of environment, posture, and general health on eyesight. The treatment is a combination of training lenses and eye exercises.

BILATERALITY The ability to use both sides of the body and brain at the same time, for example, lifting the right hand and left foot simultaneously or being able to imagine something (right brain) and write it down in words (left brain).

BIOENERGETICS A psychological and emotional healing method derived from the ideas of Wilhelm Reich. Breathing, body stress positions and observation of physical holding patterns are used to free people from their armor.

CENTRAL FIXATION, CENTRALIZATION   *see* NUCLEAR VISION

CEZANNE (1839-1906)   A French painter who extended the Impressionistic movement by creating classic solid forms from the effects of light and color.

CHAKRA   A Sanskrit word meaning revolving wheel. Chakra refers to the energy fields that correspond to seven nerve plexus along the spinal column. Each chakra is energized by one of the colors of the rainbow.

CILIARY MUSCLE   The muscle which encircles the lens of the eye. It contracts and releases. This action changes the shape of the lens producing accommodation.

CONE CELLS   The specialized nerve cells on the retina which produce color and detail vision.

CONSCIOUS   Realized awareness, perception that is known to oneself.

SUBCONSCIOUS   perceptions, realities, processes which exist but are not felt or perceived.

UNCONSCIOUS   unawareness, an action not intended. Often implies that if you had been aware you would have acted differently.

CORNEA   The transparent front of the eye that covers the iris and the pupil.

CROSS CRAWL   An integrative remedial self-help action which reaffirms the bilateral patterning laid down during the crawling stage of infancy.

DIOPTER   One diopter is the refractive power of a lens needed to focus a point of light at one metre's distance.

DYSLEXIA   A state in which the individual has 'switched off' parts of their abilities due to stress or trying too hard. This may result in slowed reading, reversal of letters when writing, or disruption of personal expressiveness.

EGO   The conscious centre of the spectrum of one's being.

FOVEA CENTRALIS   The point of keenest vision in the eye. A spot on the retina where cone cells are highly concentrated.

FUSION   The brain and mind's ability to blend together the messages coming from both eyes.

the 'GATE'   The appearance of two fingers that arises when one finger is held up close in front of the eyes and when your attention is in the distance.

the 'GREAT WHITE GLOW'   The white aura seen around letters and words when viewing black print on white paper with a relaxed mind.

HEMISPHERE   The right half or the left half of the brain.

HERBS   Annual and perennial plants used for food, medicine, seasoning, perfume. Examples are mint, comfrey, corn, cabbage, ginger, lavender.

HOMEOSTASIS   The innate tendency to maintain internal balance.

HOMOLATERAL   Using only one side of the brain. This can result in an inability to perform creatively, express spontaneously and maintain health.

HYPOGLYCEMIA   Low blood sugar. One eats something sweet and gets a short burst of energy, followed by fatigue and irritability.

HYPEROPIA   (long-sightedness) A state where the image of the close object seen falls behind the retina resulting in blur. Emotionally, an inability to be comfortable with intimate experiences. Usually compensated for by the prescribing of magnifying or 'plus' lenses.

HYPOTHALAMUS   A small area at the base of the forebrain which synthesizes hormones regulating growth, metabolism, sexual behavior, pleasure/pain and resistance to stress. The hypothalmus also controls the action of the iris and ciliary muscles.

INTEGRATION   The merging and blending of abilities and characteristics. The act of unifying rather than isolating. Denotes a state of high human ability.

IRIDOLOGY   The study and practice of discerning body conditions by observing the iris of the eye.

IRIS   The colored disc around the pupil of the eye between the cornea and lens which controls the amount of light entering the eye.

LEFT BRAIN   The left hemispere of the brain, its abilities and actions such as counting, analysing, verbalizing, reasoning, making an effort to do things.

LENS   The transparent layered curved structure that sits between the pupil and vitreous humor. The lens gently bends entering light and helps cast it upon the retina.

LENS   An optical device made of plastic or glass which brings light rays closer together or spreads them apart. Compensatory lenses are eyeglasses which bend light for unbalanced visual systems.

MACROCOSM   The universal perspective. The 'big picture'.

MICROCOSM   The 'little' world, The universe seen in miniature.

MUSCLE TESTING   Using the muscles of the body as indicators of energy supply from the brain. One puts pressure on a muscle and tests whether it remains strong or suddenly weakens. Under certain conditions such as eating white sugar, thinking negatively, sitting awkwardly, the muscle will likely weaken. Thinking positively, poised sitting, a green apple, may cause the muscle to strengthen once again.

MYOPIA (shortsightedness)   A refractive state of the visual system in which the image of distant objects fall in front of the retina, causing blur. Metaphorically, an inability to clearly perceive a large viewpoint. Usually compensated for by the prescribing of contractive 'minus' lenses.

NATURAL VISION IMPROVEMENT   A lifestyle method of improving eyesight by wholistic means without the use of optical devices. The Bates method merged with modern theories of brain function, character, and responsibility for one's self and state of being.

NEONATE   A child that's just been born.

NUCLEAR VISION   A term used in this book to represent centred, centralized, foveal vision. Mentally the object regarded is seen more clearly than anything surrounding it. Physically the light from the object regarded falls into the fovea centralis.

ORTHOPTICS   A method of exercising eye muscles to correct crossed eyes and muscular weaknesses.

PALMING   The act of gently placing the cupped palms of the hands over the closed eyes to relax the eye area while visualizing pleasant images.

PARASYMPATHETIC NERVOUS SYSTEM   That branch of the autonomic nervous sytem which takes care of relaxation and digestion. Stimulation of parasympathetic results in accommodation for near vision.

PATCHING   The act of covering one eye with an obscuring material to encourage the uncovered eye to wake up and perceive.

PATHOLOGY   A disease condition.

CATARACT   a condition where the lens of the eye becomes opaque blocking the light from reaching the retina.

GLAUCOMA   a higher than normal pressure within the eyeball.

MACULAR DEGENERATION   the nerve cells of the macula deteriorate leading to loss of central 'nuclear' vision.

RETINAL DETACHMENT   the layers of nerve cells at the back of the eye pull away from their foundation. Can occur with a severe blow to the head or with very high degrees of myopia.

PINEAL GLAND   A small cone-shaped organ at the base of the brain which may regulate the flow of sexual energy in response to sunlight cycles.

PITUITARY GLAND   The body's 'concertmaster' which secretes hormones that regulate the endocrine system. The pituitary takes its orders from the hypothalamus.

PRESBYOPIA, "OLD AGE SIGHT"   The gradual loss of accommodative powers for near vision. Compensated for by the wearing of magnifying or 'plus' lenses.

PUPIL   The circular opening in the centre of the iris which allows light to enter the interior chamber of the eye and fall up the retina.

RADIAL KERATOTOMY   A surgical practice of slitting the front of the cornea to flatten it and change the refractive state of the eye. A medical compensatory treatment for myopia.

REFRACTIVE ERROR   A deviation in the eye's ability to bend incoming light to create a clear image. Variations are labelled as hyperopia, myopia, presbyopia, astigmatism.

REICHIAN THERAPY   A way of changing human unhappiness by freeing breathing patterns and increasing the flow of biological energy through the body. Values are natural childbirth, self-regulation, positive sexual expression and human autonomy.

REPRESSING   Putting down, not allowing expression.

RETINA   The responsive layer of specialized nerve cells at the back of the eye which change light into electrical impulses and send those impulses back to the visual brain.

RETINOSCOPY   The objective examination of the refractive powers of the eye by observation with a retinoscope.

RETINOSCOPE   An optical instrument that casts a beam of light into the eye revealing whether the eye is in a state of refractive error.

RIGHT BRAIN   The right hemisphere of the brain and its abilities and action such as rhythmic movement through space, imaging, musicality, insight and supplying balanced energy to all body muscles.

ROD CELLS   The nerve cells in the retina which allow for perception of
light and dark. Stimulated in dim light, they do not register colour.

SACCADES   The quick small movements of the eye that enable the eyes to
pick up details and to move from one object of interest to another.

SCANNING   The action of moving the attention flowingly from one area
to another.

SPINDLE CELLS   The spindle cells sense the length of muscle fibres and send
messages to the brain.

SPINDLE CELL TECHNIQUE   If you shorten the muscle fibre deliberately, the
message relayed to the brain is 'This muscle is too cramped!' The
brain responds by releasing the spasm that originally arose through
conscious effort and strain. The muscle lengthens and is again under
the jurisdiction of the right, relaxing brain.

STRABISMUS, SQUINT   Turning of an eye so that both eyes are unable to
point toward the same place simultaneously.

SUPPRESSING   To hold back, keep in your urges, feelings and desires.

SUNNING   The act of relaxing in the sunlight with the eyes closed moving
easily, absorbing the light and centring the mind.

SWING   A movement of the attention and body which stimulates
parasympathetic function, soothes the mind and activates rapid
saccadic movements in the eyes.

'SWITCHER'   Someone who tends to jump into one side of the brain or the
other, losing integration.

'SWITCHING ON'   Becoming integrated, able to access and express total
ability and potential.

'TOUCH FOR HEALTH'   A system for lay people to correct and restore body
energy using muscle testing as instant feedback. Pressure points on
the body are activated to improve posture, relieve headaches,
indigestion, other 'ordinary' ailments before the underlying
imbalances result in disease.

TRANSITION (T) GLASSES   Undercorrected glasses worn by Natural
Vision Improvement students which give the eyes room for change
and allow the student to see adequately when needed for work
and leisure.

TROMBONING   The action of covering one eye with the palm and moving
an object near and far to strengthen and flex the components of
accommodation. For restoring clarity at close-point.

ULTRA-VIOLET   That part of the electromagnetic spectrum of the sun's rays
with slightly greater frequency than violet. It is also emitted by
artificial lamps that are used for healing, growing plants and
forming vitamins. Ultra-violet is said to be necessary for human
health as it stimulates the pituitary gland.

Index

1   Natural vision is mine for life.

2   Seeing is a way of being.

3   Clear sight comes when the eyes and mind are relaxed and mobile.

4   Many parts of me are active in seeing. My brain, body, mind and feelings join together in creating a coherent visual world full of color and meaning.

5   I am able to see clearly the far distant mountains which change from ruddy red to pink to violet when the sun sets. Appreciating the variety and beauty of the living earth keeps me young and enthusiastic.

6   Pluck three juicy red berries from a thorny raspberry bush and toss them into your mouth where they burst with flavor and sweetness. You'll find silvery blue huckleberries in spongy boglands. Two-inch blackberries grow on the roadsides in Washington State. They will stain your hands burgundy red.

7   Sit on one end of a fallen tree in a New England forest in autumn. A perky black-eyed chipmunk with a white stripe running down its head and back may be sitting at the other end holding a polished golden-brown acorn. Smell the spicy tang of the air as leaves flutter to the ground. Flaming orange, tawny yellow, and rusty red carpets weave themselves around you. Pick up the leaf that has gently touched your foot. Hold it up to the slanting sun and trace its veins.

8   Imagine standing on a mesa in Arizona. Look down over the faint tracery of miles of interlaced irrigation canals. Digging in the ground you uncover shards of pottery painted in geometric designs. The hot dusty wind blows into your lungs. You have a vision of people walking about. They are carrying tall jars of water, tilling rows of maize, laughing and calling to one another.

9   You might like to live the life of a wild otter. You slide down a muddy bank, splashing into the sparkling water. Play under water. Twist your sinuous body, undulate past a docile fish and a drowsy mossy green turtle.

10   Inquisitive imaginative minds lead themselves into delightful adventures.

NUCLEAR

CREATE

IMAGE

SEE

OPEN

EYE

COLOR

BEAUTY

FREEDOM

If you are able to name this size letter at 20 feet or six metres, you have approximately 20/20 or 6/6 visual acuity.

E

If you are able to name this size letter at 20 feet or six metres, you have approximately 20/40 or 6/12 vision.

E

If you are able to name this size letter at 14 inches or 36 centimetres, you have approximately 20/20 or 6/6 vision at the 'near point'.

E

If you are able to name this size letter at 14 inches or 36 centimetres, you have approximately 20/40 or 6/12 vision at the 'near point'.

E

NEAR
IS
FAR
FAR
IS
NEAR